Praise for *The Memory*

"Social interaction is beneficial for preserving cognition, as many of the most pleasurable experiences are those we share with others. Staying social is just as important as intellectual stimulation when it comes to keeping the mind nimble and Judi and Shari Zucker give valuable information in *The Memory Diet* to help us all preserve our most treasured life experiences!"

—Dr. Ava Cadell, PhD, author of *NeuroLoveology*

"Doctor Alzheimer, who first used the term 'Alzheimer's disease,' identified this brain dysfunction condition as stemming from the unhealthy animal-based western diet, which causes multiple strokes, edema, and disruption of brain waves. I believe from my 40 years of work the best way to prevent and treat dementia associated with atherosclerotic brain disorders is to adopt a plant protein diet and lifestyle medicine approach described in *The Memory Diet*."

—Nick Delgado, PhD and author of *Simply Healthy* and *Healthy Aging Breakthrough*

"Wow! I love this most needed book! With dementia and Alzheimer's at an all-time high and the number of Baby Boomers at an all time high of almost 80 million, nothing could be more important than the crucial whole plant foods that are not only the building blocks of the body (most importantly the brain first) but are our true medicine in not only reversing but healing many maladies including a starving brain! Who wouldn't love the amazing foods and recipes in this book over the often toxic medications and their side effects? Fabulous job!"

—Catie J. Wyman Norris, CNC, ND, nutritionist to the stars, author of *The Truth About Calcium* and formulator of Catie's Whole Plant Food's and Simply Young Evidence Based Whole Plant Foods

THE Memory DIET

More Than 150 Healthy Recipes for the Proper Care and Feeding of Your Brain

JUDI AND SHARI ZUCKER

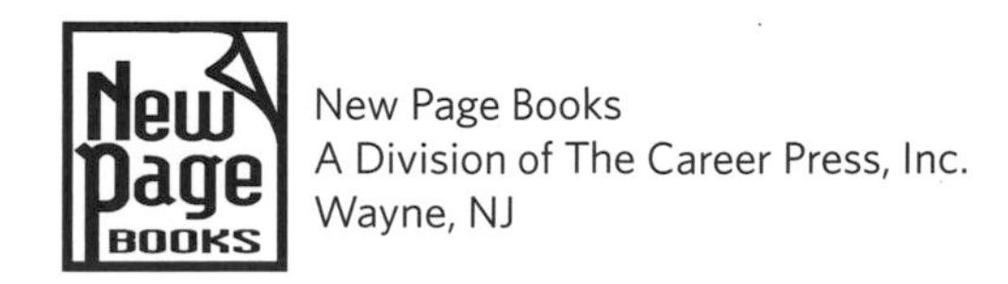
New Page Books
A Division of The Career Press, Inc.
Wayne, NJ

Copyright © 2016 by Judi and Shari Zucker

All rights reserved under the Pan-American and International Copyright Conventions. This book may not be reproduced, in whole or in part, in any form or by any means electronic or mechanical, including photocopying, recording, or by any information storage and retrieval system now known or hereafter invented, without written permission from the publisher, The Career Press.

THE MEMORY DIET
EDITED BY JODI BRANDON
TYPESET BY PERFECTYPE, NASHVILLE, TENN.
Printed in the U.S.A.

To order this title, please call toll-free 1-800-CAREER-1 (NJ and Canada: 201-848-0310) to order using VISA or MasterCard, or for further information on books from Career Press.

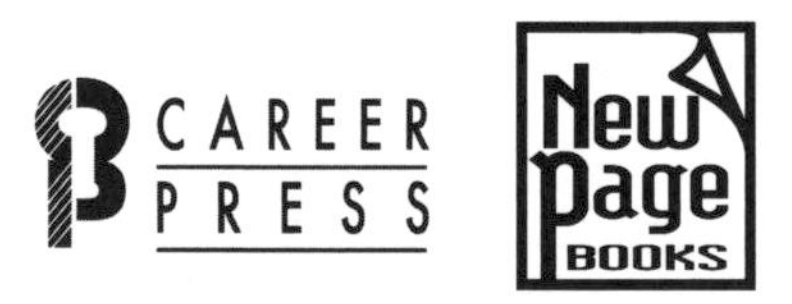

The Career Press, Inc.
12 Parish Drive
Wayne, NJ 07470
www.careerpress.com
www.newpagebooks.com

Library of Congress Cataloging-in-Publication Data

CIP Data Available Upon Request.

DEDICATION

We would like to dedicate this book to our mother, who has dementia. She inspired us to write this book so we could help those suffering from memory loss and those who want to prevent it. We have learned to never underestimate the value of a memory. We love you, Mom!

ACKNOWLEDGMENTS

We would like to thank our family and friends for their support and love.

We would like to thank our editors, Lauren Manoy, Jodi Brandon, and Gina Schenck for their organizational abilities and attention to detail. For their input on this project, we would like to acknowledge everyone at Career Press/New Page Books. Special thanks to Adam Schwartz, Michael Pye, and Laurie Kelly-Pye for their support and helpful suggestions.

Thank you, Jill Marsal, our literary agent, for your guidance and professional expertise.

We are grateful to be twins and share our passion to educate others on the benefits of a healthful lifestyle. It's great to be PIFs (partners in fun)!

CONTENTS

FOREWORD

With our population of aging individuals ever-increasing, we have come to realize the serious nature of memory impairment. In the past, we accepted memory loss in the elderly as unavoidable. However, despite increased age having some impact on our ability to remember, science has shown that many types of cognitive impairment and memory loss can be successfully treated, reversed, and even prevented.

Simple steps like eating well, getting enough sleep, decreasing stress, not smoking, minimizing alcohol intake, taking nutritional supplements, exercising, and keeping your brain active can help prevent dementia. Why the emphasis on food? Simply, the Standard American Diet (aptly named "SAD" for short) is full of processed foods, sugars, simple carbohydrates, and trans fats that are responsible for many serious health problems that can include impairment of mental acuity, weight gain, heart disease, chronic inflammation, and hormonal imbalances.

So, one of the most important things you can do is adopt a healthy, well-balanced diet, which can have a profound effect on your cognitive function and memory. Judi and Shari Zucker are strong believers in the connection between good health and nutritious dietary habits. In *The Memory Diet* they present a treasure trove of recipes that focus on foods that are good both for the brain and overall health.

Based on the latest research on brain health, Judi and Shari share tasty recipes that focus on a plant-based diet low in sugar and "bad" fats, and high in flavor. They have created easy and delicious meals, which center around fruits, vegetables, legumes, whole grains, and nuts. These foods are also known to help prevent cardiovascular disease by enhancing overall blood circulation, which also supports your brain function. In addition, the antioxidant-rich fruits and vegetables help protect your brain and other cells from oxidizing or "rusting," just as iron rusts when exposed to moisture. Then, many plant-based foods such as avocados and nuts contain healthy fats needed to form healthy cell membranes, especially in the brain, which is almost 70 percent fat.

Read on to find out how you can eat your way to a longer, healthier life, and one where you can keep your mental faculties operating optimally for many years.

—Hyla Cass, MD, author of *8 Weeks to Vibrant Health*
www.cassmd.com

PREFACE

It was a beautiful December day in Los Angeles, and a family tradition was to walk to the Beverly Hills Hotel and see the festive decorations. Our mother had store credit at the hotel, and we were waiting for her to get it. She frantically looked at us and said she couldn't find the credit slip. We laughed and said to her, "You will find it." She had a frightened look on her face and sternly said to us, "I am scared that I forgot where I put the credit slip. I am really scared!" At the time we didn't realize that she had been experiencing bouts of forgetfulness. Our mother began to forget many things and she was worried. We made an appointment to see a brain doctor, and the doctor ran several tests. The results showed that our mother had dementia—specifically semantic dementia, a variance of Alzheimer's. The doctor told us that our mother's form of dementia was not genetic but environmentally induced. Knowing our mother, her dementia could have been caused by many things, such as her longtime use of sleeping pills, alcohol, sugar, or processed foods, or the multiple surgeries she had with anesthesia. Although we were told we could not reverse her dementia, at least it was worth a try to slow it down and do whatever we could to preserve her memory! Whether it's a family member or you being diagnosed with a memory disorder, it can be overwhelming. There is hope, and with simple lifestyle changes you can decrease your chances of getting a memory disorder and preserving the memory you deserve to have. In *The Memory Diet*, we share what we learned about maintaining brain health, and we share our favorite tasty, brain-boosting recipes!

INTRODUCTION

According to the World Health Organization there are more than 47 million people living with dementia and that number is projected to increase to 75.6 million by 2030.[1] A new case of dementia is diagnosed every four seconds.[2] Unfortunately, our mother is one of the many people living with dementia. When we found out our mother had been diagnosed with dementia we were devastated! We were determined to do whatever we could to help our mother. We did extensive research on brain health, and we have successfully helped our mother slow down her memory loss. We are committed to helping others understand cognitive decline, and how to prevent and deal with it. Through our research we have created tasty, brain-boosting recipes that everyone can enjoy! In *The Memory Diet* we provide current, valuable, and scientific-based information about memory loss, as well as delicious brain healthy recipes!

The Memory Diet centers around the MIND diet, which stands for Mediterranean Intervention Neurodegenerative Delay. The MIND diet originated from a study at Rush University Medical Center and is a hybrid of the Mediterranean diet and the Dietary Approaches to Stop Hypertension (DASH) diet. According to the MIND Diet Study this diet plan may reduce the risk of developing Alzheimer's by as much as 53 percent.[3] *The Memory Diet* focuses on the plant-based recommendations of the MIND diet. These plant-based foods center around green leafy vegetables, nuts, berries, beans, whole grains, and olive oil. The MIND diet does include fish and chicken once a week. However, those nutrients that help the brain found in fish and chicken can be found in plant sources that we share in *The Memory Diet*. For example, DHA and omega-3s found in fish can be found in flaxseeds, chia seeds, walnuts, and marine algae that are healthier for the body as they do not contain mercury, which is commonly found in fish.

The MIND diet recommends avoiding the following foods: red meat, butter, cheese, pastries, and fried foods. Researchers found that even those who didn't stick to the diet perfectly but followed it "moderately well" reduced their risk of Alzheimer's by about a third. Furthermore, the study, published in the journal *Alzheimer's & Dementia*, looked at more than 900 people between the ages of 58 to 98 who filled out food questionnaires and underwent repeated neurological testing.[4] It found participants whose diets most closely followed the MIND recommendations had a level of cognitive function that equivalent of a person 7.5 years younger![5]

A plant-based diet that includes leafy greens, vegetables, berries, nuts, beans, and whole grains slows down and prevents cognitive decline. There are more than 150 tasty, plant-based recipes in *The Memory Diet* that are all free of white refined sugar, processed foods, and gluten. In *The Memory Diet* no refined sugars are used because insulin resistance, basically "sugar intolerance," is being proven in research to be the underlying cause of many of our modern diseases, such as neurological diseases like Alzheimer's and many forms of cancer, besides obvious problems such as diabetes. The recipes found in this book nourish the brain and body!

The recipes taste great, too! After all, even the most nutritious foods aren't beneficial if no one eats them. That is why you will find that the dishes in this book—soups and salads, smoothies and snacks, as well as entrees, side dishes, and desserts—are tasty and satisfying.

It is important to eat foods that are good for the brain, and it is equally important to eat foods that are cooked correctly to minimize memory loss. In *The Memory Diet* dishes that require cooking are cooked on a low heat. This is crucial to making foods healthier for the brain. *The Memory Diet* addresses AGEs (advanced glycation end products). AGEs in the diet represent pathogenic compounds that have been linked to the induction and progression of many chronic diseases including Alzheimer's disease.

AGEs reinforce previous observations that high temperature and low moisture consistently can strongly drive AGE formation in foods, whereas comparatively brief heating time, low temperatures, high moisture, and/or pre-exposure to an acidified environment (using lemon or vinegar when cooking) are effective strategies to limit new AGE formation in food. The potentially negative effects of traditional forms of cooking and food processing have typically remained outside the realm of health considerations. However, accumulation of AGEs due to the systematic heating and processing of foods offers a new explanation for adverse health effects. *The Memory Diet* focuses on low-AGE-generating cooking methods such as steaming, stewing, and boiling. Animal-derived foods that are high in fat and protein such as meat and poultry are generally AGE-rich and prone to new AGE formation during cooking. In contrast, carbohydrate-rich foods such as vegetables, fruits, and whole grains contain relatively few AGEs, even after cooking. The formation of new AGEs during cooking was prevented by the AGE-inhibitory compound aminoguanidine and significantly reduced cooking with moist heat, using shorter cooking times, and cooking at lower temperatures (250 degrees or lower), and by the use of acidic ingredients such as lemon or apple cider vinegar.

A study completed by the Icahn School of Medicine at Mount Sinai Hospital showed that a diet high in glycotoxins (AGEs) found in high concentration in well-done meat is a risk factor in developing age-related dementia. The study, titled "Oral Glycotoxins Are Modifiable Cause of Dementia and the Metabolic Syndrome in Mice and Humans," was published in the *Journal Proceedings of the National Academy of Science (PNAS)*; *Alzheimer's News Today* reported the study.[6]

In the study, mice that were on a diet high in glycotoxins called advanced glycation end products (AGEs), were found to have significantly higher likelihood of developing dementia-like symptoms. They also had greater levels of amyloid beta proteins—the basis of "brain plaque" in Alzheimer's patients—in their brains.

The research team assessed AGEs in blood samples from 93 individuals who were over 60 years in age for a nine-month period. Data on the participants' cognitive function and eating habits, especially of food products rich in glycotoxins, were analyzed. The insulin sensitivity of each participant was also determined, as it represents a major biomarker for metabolic syndromes, including obesity and diabetes. Similar to the results in mice, participants with higher blood levels of AGEs experienced more cognitive decline and a reduction in insulin sensitivity, suggesting that regular consumption of AGEs in overcooked food may lead to diabetes and obesity. The team concluded that food-derived AGEs are a modifiable risk factor for both metabolic syndrome disorders and Alzheimer's disease, and suggested that an AGE-restricted diet may provide an effective therapeutic strategy for both disorders.

The Memory Diet provides foods recommended in the MIND diet, has more than 150 plant-based, brain-healthy recipes, and includes a 7-Day Memory Meal plan. *The Memory Diet* has brain-worthy dishes that take in account AGEs and implements safe cooking methods to ensure lower AGEs for the body. Dishes that require heating are not fried or "browned"; instead they are steamed or baked at heat not exceeding 250 degrees F.

In *The Memory Diet* we share what is and isn't normal memory loss, and how lifestyle choices can make a huge difference in a healthful brain. We share how to stock a mindful kitchen, and provide healthy food options that include organic, GMO-free (genetically modified) foods, and supplements for cognitive health. There is an extensive resources section of informative Websites, organizations, and reliable manufacturers that support a brain-healthy lifestyle.

CHAPTER 1

About Your Memory: Maintaining Memory Health

With dementia on the rise, it's easy to become paranoid when you forget something. However, memory loss is not an inevitable part of the aging process, and it's important to distinguish between what's normal when it comes to memory loss and when you should be concerned. Most of us have experienced forgetting where we put our keys or cell phone, or have forgotten an acquaintance's name. Normal forgetfulness is more common in older adults. Some examples of normal forgetfulness are not remembering the name of an actor in a movie you just saw, or standing in the middle of your kitchen and suddenly blanking on what you wanted to write on your grocery list. In most cases if we wait a few minutes the information will come to mind. Memory lapses can be frustrating, but most of the time they are not cause for concern. As we age we experience physiological changes that can cause glitches in the way our brain functions. It can take longer to learn and recall information. Taking longer to do something does not equate to serious memory loss.

Dementia is a general term for a decline in mental ability severe enough to interfere with daily life. Memory loss is an example of dementia. Dementia is not a specific disease, as it describes a wide range of symptoms associated with a decline in memory. There are many forms of dementia, which include vascular and mixed dementia. Alzheimer's disease is the most common type of dementia. Dementia can be overwhelming for the people who have it, and also for their families and caregivers. If you or someone you love is experiencing any signs of a more serious memory problem, then it's important to see a doctor to find the root of the cause.

Memory loss does not automatically mean that you have dementia. There are many reasons why you may be experiencing memory problems, which may include any of the following: stress, depression, hearing or vision loss, thyroid problems, genetic propensity, past head injury, stoke, drug use, or vitamin deficiencies. Even if you are not displaying the common symptoms of dementia, it is always a good idea to take steps to prevent a small problem from becoming a large problem!

It is true that as we age, the body does break down, and normal memory loss or forgetfulness can occur. Age is one of the factors that may increase your chances of getting Alzheimer's as most of the cases occur after the age of 65. The primary difference between age-related memory loss and dementia is that age-related memory loss has little impact on your daily performance and ability to do what you want to do. However, dementia is marked by a persistent decline in two or more intellectual abilities, such as memory, language, judgment, and abstract thinking. Severe memory loss disrupts your work, hobbies, social activities, and family relationships.

Fortunately, the brain is capable of producing new brain cells at any age and memory loss does not have to happen. Keeping the brain sharp is important. Your lifestyle choices, health habits, and daily activities have a huge impact on the health of your brain. The good news is that many mental abilities are largely not affected by normal aging, such as your ability to do things you have always done and continue to do often, your wisdom and knowledge you have acquired from life experiences, and your innate common sense and ability to reason. Making smart lifestyle choices can decrease and possibly prevent your chances of getting many diseases including dementia.

Maintaining Memory Health

For many years many of us have been under the impression that there is little we can do to prevent Alzheimer's disease or dementia, and that memory loss is part of the natural progression of aging. It seems like all we can do is hope for the best and wait for a cure. Alzheimer's drugs have not shown much benefit, which underscores the importance of prevention throughout your lifetime. Studies have shown that lifestyle choices such as eating right, exercising, staying mentally and socially active, keeping stress in check, getting adequate sleep, and taking certain supplements can reduce your risk of getting memory loss. By leading a brain healthy lifestyle, you can be able to prevent Alzheimer's symptoms and slow down or even reverse the process of deterioration.[1]

In this chapter we will discuss the impact of lifestyle choices and how they can prevent dementia. We will also discuss the lifestyle choices to avoid in preventing your chances of getting dementia.

Exercise

Exercise is critical in preventing dementia. According to the Alzheimer's Research and Prevention Foundation, physical exercise reduces your risk of developing Alzheimer's disease by 50 percent.[2] The *New York Times* health and science writer Gretchen Reynalds wrote, "Exercise potentially does more to bolster thinking than thinking does."[3]

People who get regular, vigorous exercise also tend to stay mentally sharp in their 70s and 80s. Exercising is good for the lungs, and people whose memories and mental acuity remain strong in old age characteristically have good lung function. Exercise helps reduce the risk for diabetes, high cholesterol, high blood pressure, and stroke. These are all illnesses that lead to memory loss. Most importantly, animal research has shown that exercise increases the level of neurotropins, substances in the body that nourish brain cells and help protect them against damage from stroke and other injuries.[4] Exercise can trigger a change in the way the amyloid precursor protein in the brain is metabolized, thus slowing down the onset and progression of Alzheimer's. It also increases levels of a protein known as Peroxisome proliferator-activator-activated receptor-gamma coactivator (PGC-1 alpha), a protein that is helpful to the brain. People with Alzheimer's have less PGC-1 alpha in their brains, and cells that contain more of the protein produce less of the toxic amyloid protein associated with Alzheimer's.

Exercise doesn't need to be extreme, but should be regular. The Centers of Disease Control (CDC) and the American College of Sports Medicine (ACSM) recommend that adults get about two and a half hours (150 minutes) of moderate-intensity aerobic activity each week.[5,6] Moderate-intensity aerobic activity is defined as movement that raises your heart rate and makes you break a sweat. An easy way to tell whether your exertion level is moderate is that you will be able to talk, but not sing, while exercising.

Here are some ways to get daily exercise:

» When possible, walk instead of driving or riding.
» Use the stairs instead of taking the elevator.
» Exercise at home, possibly with an exercise video.
» Plant a garden.
» Take an exercise class or join a health club.
» Swim regularly, if you have access to a pool, lake, or beach.
» Learn a sport that requires modest physical exertion, such as tennis.
» Dance while listening to music.

Playing ping pong, also known as table tennis, is known to improve one's attention and concentration. Japanese researchers also found that in players older than 50, ping pong improved brain function by activating specific neurons. It showed promise in preventing dementia as well.[7]

Exercise helps boost your energy levels, helps you control your weight, strengthens your muscles and bones, and decreases your chances of developing type 2 diabetes and cancers of the breast, colon, and prostate. Exercise stimulates the growth of brain cells and protects against brain cell death. The University of British Columbia finds that regular aerobic exercise can actually increase the size of your hippocampus (the part of your brain that helps you learn and remember).[8] Basically, exercise increases your general quality of life and decreases your chances of experiencing memory loss.

Exercise may include many types of movement from running to bicycling. When doing a sport that may be more dangerous, such as bicycling or football, we highly recommend you wear protective gear such as a helmet to avoid head injuries. A Tufts University study found that even a single trauma to the brain could lead to Alzheimer's.[9] Even being aware of your surroundings to avoid falling or injuries is a good idea. It's important to nail down rugs, dry slippery floors promptly, make sure your stairs have sturdy handrails, and avoid using step-stools or ladders without someone spotting you. Wearing the right fitting shoes is important, too, because the height of the heel can affect your balance, which can cause you to fall.

New research indicates music can help those with dementia. Researchers at the Institute for Music and Neurologic Function at Beth Abraham Family of Health Services in New York state claim there is a biological link between the auditory cortex of the brain and its limbic system (where emotions are processed) that make it possible for sound to be processed almost immediately by the areas associated with long-term memory and emotions.[10] Music often has a personal significance to someone and is connected with historical events that engage a happy response from those with dementia. One of the noted neurologists, Dr. Oliver Sacks, states that people with neurological damage learned to move better, remember more, and even regain speech through listening to and playing music.[11] In numerous clinical studies of older people with Alzheimer's and other forms of dementia, familiar music, not medication, has reduced depression, lessened agitation, increased sociability, movement, and cognitive ability, and decreased problem behaviors often associated with dementia.[12] Published in *Science Translation Medicine*, researchers from the University of Queensland in Australia, are finding that a particular type of ultrasound called a focused therapeutic ultrasound, which incorporates noninvasive beams of sound waves into the brain tissue, has been able to stimulate the microglial cells in the brain to activate.[13] Microglia cells are basically the resident macrophages of the brain and spinal cord, and act as the first and main form of active immune defense in the central nervous system (CNS). Macrophages are a type of white blood cell that engulfs and digests cellular debris or foreign substances such as cancer cells. They are able to clear out the toxic beta-amyloid clumps that are responsible for the worst symptoms of Alzheimer's.

We can tell you firsthand that our mother's greatest joy is to listen to music! It makes her happy, and she loves to listen to it when she goes walking every day. We definitely believe the joy she gets from listening to music combined with her daily exercise has slowed down her dementia considerably.

Staying Mentally and Socially Active

Physical activity is essential to maintaining your mental health, and so is mental exercising. Reading regularly, keeping up with current affairs, learning a new hobby, learning how to play a new instrument, playing challenging games, and learning a new language are all activities that keep the mind active. According to research done at Singapore Management University, learning a foreign language can help your brain process information better and help you focus more sharply.[14] Whether it is learning a new language or doing word games, these activities can delay and help decrease the onset of dementia.

People who have spent more time in formal education appear to have a lower incidence of mental decline, even when they have brain abnormalities. Researchers believe that education may help your brain develop a stronger nerve cell network that compensates for nerve cell damage caused by Alzheimer's.[15] Advance education may help keep memory strong by getting people into the habit of being mentally active. Regardless of your level of education, anyone can be an active, lifelong learner. Some people continue their education with adult education classes or advanced degrees even in late adulthood. Mental stimulation, especially learning something new, such as learning to play an instrument, getting a new iPhone or computer, or learning a new language, is associated with a decreased risk of Alzheimer's. Researchers suspect that mental challenge helps to build up your brain, making it less susceptible to the lesions associated with Alzheimer's disease.[16]

Mental exercises include social interaction. A diverse and widely developed network is just as important as intellectual stimulation when it comes to keeping your mind nimble. It is vital to regularly stay in touch with friends and family. Maintaining social interaction is beneficial for preserving cognition, and many of the most pleasurable experiences are those you share with others. Regularly schedule any activity you enjoy. A visit to the theater, a walk in the park, anything that involves interaction with other people, joining a group or class, doing volunteer work or getting a job, and playing team sports are all great ways to stay socially active and important in keeping the brain healthy.

Getting the Proper Amount of Sleep

Sleep is essential for memory health as well as overall health. Although people vary widely in their individual sleep needs, research suggests that six to eight hours of sleep per night is ideal.[17] The quality of your sleep may be even more important than the amount of sleep. Breathing problems during sleep, such as obstructive sleep apnea, can affect the brain. Getting a good night's sleep for some people is easier said than done, especially because insomnia becomes more common with age. However, certain habits can help. Here are some tips for better sleep:

» Turn off all lights before going to bed. One of the biggest contributors to collective sleep problems is the use of artificial light and electronics at night. Modern light bulbs and electronic devices (especially computer monitors, tablets, and cell phones) produce large amounts of blue light that "trick" our brains into thinking it is daytime.[18]

» Establish and maintain a consistent sleep schedule and routine. Go to bed at the same time each night and wake up at the same time each morning. A set sleep routine will "train" you to fall asleep and wake up more easily.

» Plan to do your most vigorous exercise early in the day. Exercising in the hours immediately before bedtime causes physiological changes that interfere with sleep. Exercising in the morning, on the other hand, enhances your alertness when you need it most—at the beginning of the day.

» Avoid coffee and other sources of caffeine, such as chocolate, many soft drinks, some brands of aspirin, and many types of teas, after mid-morning, because caffeine is a stimulant that can keep you awake for hours afterward.

» Sleep if you are tired. Trying to sleep when you are not tired has you tossing and turning all night. If you are still awake after 20 minutes in bed, get up and read for a while to help yourself relax.

- » If you experience persistent sleep problems, consult your physician so that you can find out what's wrong and get treatment if needed.

Stress Management

Stress that is chronic can take a heavy toll on the brain, leading to shrinkage in a key memory area of the brain known as the hippocampus. Stress also hampers nerve cell growth, and increases your risk of Alzheimer's disease and dementia. Here are some simple techniques that can help keep your stress levels in check:

- » Breathe! Stress alters your breathing rate and impacts oxygen levels in the brain. Quite simple and free!
- » Schedule daily relaxation activities. Keeping stress under control is not that hard. When you schedule your daily activities have fun making a to-do list and write it in the color red. A study from the University of Regensburg in Germany found that the color red "binds" into our memory better than other colors. It's an ideal color for recalling what is on your to-do list.[19]
- » Make relaxation a priority, whether it's a walk in the park, playtime with your dog, yoga, or a soothing bath.
- » While relaxing you might close your eyes to remember something great that happened that day. Research from the University of Surrey in the UK found that closing your eyes while recalling an event could help you remember details 23 percent more accurately.[20] It is believed that once visual distractions are removed, your brain focuses more efficiently.
- » Regular meditation, prayer, reflection, and religious practice may immunize you against the damaging effects of stress.
- » Be positive. Studies show that optimists tend to have increased lifespans, more responsive immune systems, and a lower risk of cardiovascular disease. Make a point to regularly ask yourself, "What if everything went right instead of

wrong?" Positive thinking can actually activate the physical ability of your brain to adapt and change.

Supplements for Brain Health

It is not always possible to get all the nutrients you need through diet alone. Modern agricultural practices have leached vital minerals from our cropland. Fruits and vegetables grown in this depleted soil do not have enough nutrients. Nutrients begin to decline the minute a plant is picked. Cold storage continues the destruction of nutrient content, too. In an ideal world, we would be able to eat all our food within an hour of harvesting, but this not possible. Therefore it is important to supplement the diet with vitamins, minerals, and herbs to reduce cognitive decline. Because there are so many supplements that can boost your memory and cognitive function, it can be confusing to know which ones to take. However, certain supplements have shown promise in preventing dementia. For example, a study published in the *Proceedings of the National Academy of Sciences* found that vitamin B6, B12, and folic acid may help slow the progression of Alzheimer's disease.[21] Vitamin D, magnesium, and omega-3 fatty acid (DHA) are believed to preserve and improve brain health, too. Vitamin E, ginkgo biloba, coenzyme Q10, curcumin (the plant chemical found in the root of turmeric), Acetyl-L-carnitine, probiotics, resveratrol, aloe vera juice, spirulina, alpha-lipoic acid (ALA), phosphatidylserine (PS), Ashwagandha root, and vinpocetine may all be beneficial in the prevention or delay of Alzheimer's and dementia symptoms. It is important to choose supplements that are natural and not synthetic. Natural forms tend to be more active and easier to absorb than synthetic versions.

In general, B vitamins help your body transform food into energy. B vitamins lower homocysteine (an amino acid), which is linked to dementia. B vitamins are found in enriched grains, beans, dark leafy veggies, papayas, oranges, and cantaloupe. They also help produce red blood cells. Red blood cells are essential for good cognition and memory by helping stabilize brain chemistry. Certain vitamins are especially beneficial to the brain: B1 (thiamine), B3 (niacin), B6 (pyridoxine), B9 (folic acid or folate), B12 (cobalamin), choline, and nicotinamide adenine dinucleotide (NAD). Because the composition of B complex vitamins varies from brand to brand, it is important to follow the recommended dosage on the label.

There is a strong link between low levels of vitamin D in Alzheimer's patients and poor outcomes on cognitive tests. Researchers believe that optimal vitamin D levels may enhance the amount of important chemicals in the brain and protect brain cells by increasing the effectiveness of the glial cells that help repair damaged neurons.[22] Vitamin D may also exert some of its beneficial effects on Alzheimer's through its anti-inflammatory and immune-boosting properties. Sufficient vitamin D is imperative for proper functioning of your immune system to combat inflammation, which is also associated with Alzheimer's.

Magnesium binds to and activates more than 300 different enzymes, making it an essential ingredient for the majority of biochemical reactions in the body. Magnesium fights inflammations, enhances the utilization of antioxidants, and helps maintain the function of nerve cells. Studies show that blood concentrations of magnesium are considerably lower in patients with Alzheimer's disease than in non-Alzheimer's subjects.[23] Studies also show that magnesium supplements can help combat insomnia and cardiovascular disease, two independent risk factors for cognitive decline.[24]

DHA (docoshexaenoic acid) is found alongside another omega-3 fatty acid called EPA (eicosapentaenoic acid). It is an integral part of brain tissue and is found in high concentrations in the hippocampus. The hippocampus is the memory center of the brain. Low levels of DHA are associated with development of learning disorders in children and Alzheimer's disease in older populations. A diet rich in DHA can decrease the risk of developing mild cognitive impairment between 19 and 75 percent.[25] DHA also helps with depression. Depression is a risk factor for cognitive decline. Most supplements of DHA are from cold-water fish. However, we recommend using the vegetarian source for DHA made from seaweed. Most fish supplements are contaminated with mercury. As this is a plant-based-diet book, we advocate healthier alternatives to fish supplements. Most adults would benefit from supplementing omega-3 fatty acids daily.

Vitamin E is actually a group of eight different fat-soluble vitamins that act as powerful antioxidants, protecting your body and brain from damage caused by free radicals. A study published in *Archives of*

Neurology in 2002 suggests that vitamin E slows the rate of age-related mental decline.[26] The study looked at 2,889 people ages 65 and older who did not have dementia or other cognitive illness. Researchers asked the participants what they ate and which vitamins and mineral supplements they took, and then traced their mental function over three years. Mental function was assessed with modified mini-mental state examinations and other standard tests. Participants who consumed the most vitamin E had 36 percent less mental decline than did people who consumed the least amount of vitamin E. It's best to take natural vitamin E that contains a combination of different tocopherols and tocotrienols (the two main subgroups of vitamin E).

Gingko biloba has positive effects on dementia. Gingko, which is derived from a tree native to Asia, has long been used medicinally in China and other countries. A 1997 study from the *Journal of the American Medical Association* showed clear evidence that gingko improves performance and social functioning for those suffering from dementia.[27] Another study in 2006 found gingko as effective as the dementia drug Aricept (donepezil) for treating mild to moderate Alzheimer's type dementia.[28]

Coenzyme Q10 is a fat-soluble nutrient, the primary function of which is to help produce cellular energy, providing your body and brain with energy they need to run at optimal levels. Coenzyme Q10 is also known to be excellent for the heart.

Curcumin is helpful in almost all age-related neurological diseases. It is anti-inflammatory, an antioxidant, supports good blood sugar control, and protects the cardiovascular system against oxidative damage that leads to heart attacks and strokes.

Acetyl-L-carnitine is a derivative of the amino acid carnitine. In addition to its function as an antioxidant, acetyl-L-carnitine slows the rate at which your neurotransmitter receptors degenerate, increases oxygen availability and respiratory efficiency, and helps convert stored body fat into energy.

Probiotics are beneficial bacteria that are necessary to maintain good health. They help treat irritable bowel syndrome, infectious diarrhea, and some skin conditions, and they aid in oral health. A study out of Leiden Institute of Brain and Cognition at Leiden University in the Netherlands suggests that probiotics may actually aid in improving mood. Researchers examined 40 healthy young adults who had no mood disorders. Half of them consumed a powerful probiotic supplement every night for four weeks. The probiotic supplement was called Ecologic Barrier and contained eight types of bacteria, including Bifidobacterium, Lactobacillus, and Lactococcus. (These three types of bacteria have been shown in the past to mitigate anxiety and depression.) The other half of the participants took a placebo, although they thought they were taking probiotics. The people who took probiotic supplements began to see improvement in their moods, and they reported less reactivity to sad moods than those who took placebos. Basically the people who took probiotics supplements were better able to overcome sad moods than the others, and thus had fewer depressive thoughts. The findings shed light on the potential of probiotics to serve as a preventive therapy for depression.[29] Depression is one of the factors that can lead to Alzheimer's disease.

Resveratrol is a powerful antioxidant found in grapes, blueberries, cranberries, peanuts, and pistachios. Some people recommend drinking red wine because it contains resveratrol, but we do not advocate any alcohol consumption. Better sources of resveratrol are grapes, grape juice, grapeseed extract, and green tea extract and supplements. Resveratrol helps prevent heart disease and may prevent some kinds of cancer. Resveratrol may slow cognitive decline by preventing amyloid accumulation. It appears to have as positive impact on specific proteins called sirtuins that are known to prevent neurodegeneration. Resveratrol also lowers the blood glucose level in type 2 diabetes and reduces the bad cholesterol (LDL) and increases the good cholesterol (HDL). Studies show that having type 2 diabetes is a major risk for Alzheimer's disease.[30]

Pure aloe vera juice (or gel) has many health benefits. It is rich in vitamins B12, B1, B2, A, E, and C, niacin, and folic acid. These vitamins are required for proper brain function. Aloe vera effectively lowers the bad cholesterol (LDL) and total triglycerides, also. It accelerates the supply of blood and purifies it at the same time. This accelerates the delivery of oxygen to the organs in the body including the brain.

Spirulina is a type of blue-green algae that grows naturally in lakes with high pH and is cultivated in controlled ponds for human consumption. Potential benefits of the spirulina-rich diet include improved immune function, reduced inflammation, and disease prevention. Spirulina may even improve brain function and memory. It contains high amounts of beta-carotene, B vitamins, iron, amino acids, phytonutrients, and antioxidants. In addition to reducing inflammation in the body tissues, it can decrease inflammation of the brain. Researchers at the University of South Florida College of Medicine conducted a study on the efficiency of spirulina to protect against neurodegenerative diseases such as Parkinson's.[31] The results support the use of spirulina as a preventative supplementation. In addition, it may prevent memory loss by reducing oxidative stress in the brain, according to a study published in the *Journal of Nutritional Science and Vitaminology*.[32]

Alpha-lipoic acid (ALA) can stabilize cognitive functions among Alzheimer's and may slow the progression of the disease. Alpha-lipoic acid, also known as lipoic acid or a-lipoid acid, is a nutrient that is both fat and water soluble. It stimulates the generation of new nerve fibers on your neurons, helping to strengthen memory and slow brain aging. It is an antioxidant found in spinach, broccoli, tomatoes, peas, and Brussels sprouts. None of these sources provide enough ALA to really make a difference, so it's best to supplement your diet with ALA.

Phosphatidylserine (PS) is a phospholipid that occurs naturally in the brain. It encourages cell-to-cell communication by increasing the production of several important neurotransmitters, including acetylcholine, serotonin, epinephrine, norepinephrine, and dopamine.

Ashwagandha root (*Withania somnifera*) is an herb that is found in India, Pakistan, and Sri Lanka. It is best known for its capacity to improve resistance to emotional and physical stress, which is a common source of cognitive decline.

Vinpocetine is an extract derived from the periwinkle plant. It acts as an anti-inflammatory agent and increases blood circulation within the brain by acting as a blood thinner and dilating (widening) blood vessels.

In order to maintain great cognitive health, it is vital to know certain factors that increase your chances of getting dementia or Alzheimer's disease. It is best to avoid anesthesia, toxic chemicals that leach into our foods such as mercury and aluminum, flu vaccinations, anticholinergic or statin drugs, sleeping pills, diet pills, various prescription drugs, alcohol, sugar, processed foods, salty foods, meat, and all forms of smoking.

Prescription drugs cause more than 100,000 deaths per year and cause 1.9 million people to experience side effects so severe that they must be hospitalized.[33] Adverse drug reactions are now the fourth leading cause of death in the United States.[34] Every medication carries some risks, and memory loss is a very common side effect. Related research, presented at the annual congress of European Society of Anesthesiology (ESA), suggests that being exposed to general anesthesia can increase the risk of dementia in the elderly by as much as 35 percent.[35]

Dental amalgam fillings, which are 50-percent mercury by weight, are one of the major sources of heavy metal toxicity. Most dentists can remove the amalgams safely. Mercury can also be found in fish, which is often recommended as "brain food" because of its omega-3s. Unfortunately, most fish contains too much mercury and should be avoided.

Try to avoid aluminum. Aluminum can be found in antiperspirants, nonstick cookware, and flu vaccinations. Unfortunately, most flu vaccinations contain both mercury and aluminum, which are both well-known neurotoxic and immunotoxic agents.

Avoid anticholinergic and statin drugs. One thing to note is that most drugs that start with the prefix *anti* (such as antihistamines, antidepressants, antipsychotics, antibiotics, antispasmodics, and antihypertensives) are likely to negatively affect your acetylcholine level. Acetylcholine is the primary neurotransmitter involved with memory and learning. When one is low in acetylcholine, one becomes forgetful and has trouble concentrating. Acetylcholine deficiencies are associated with dementia and Alzheimer's disease. There are five drugs that block acetylcholine, a nervous system neurotransmitter, that have shown to increase your risk of dementia: certain nighttime pain reliever antihistamines (such as Benadryl), sleep aids, certain antidepressants, medications to control incontinence, and certain narcotic pain relievers. Antihistamines in particular also appear to reduce the absorption of vitamin B12 in the stomach, and B12 is vital for nervous system function.

Statin drugs are particularly problematic because they suppress the synthesis of cholesterol, deplete your brain of coenzyme Q10 and neurotransmitter precursors, and prevent adequate delivery of essential fatty acids and fat-soluble antioxidants to your brain by inhibiting the production of the indispensable carrier biomolecule known as low-density lipoprotein. The book *The Great Cholesterol Myth* states that these cholesterol-lowering medications might be the single worst group of drugs for the brain.[36] One quarter of your brain is made up of cholesterol. Cholesterol is necessary for memory, learning, and fast thinking. Statin drugs are cellular poisons that accelerate aging and promote muscle fatigue, diabetes, and memory loss and unfortunately, these cholesterol lowering drugs have a negative effect on the brain and can lead to disastrous side effects.

Sleeping pills can increase your chances of getting dementia. Prescription sleeping pills are notorious for causing memory loss. Some people refer to the popular drug Ambien as "the amnesia drug." It is not unusual for some users to experience night terrors, sleep walking, sleep driving, and hallucinations. Prescription sleeping pills can put you in a state similar to being passed-out drunk or in a coma while bypassing the restorative sleep your brain needs. Sleeping well is vital to brain health and makes a challenging day feel a little less daunting.

Drinking alcohol and binge drinking are both linked to stroke and dementia. In fact, people who reported consuming more than five bottles of beer in one sitting, or one bottle of wine, in midlife were three times as likely as non-binge drinkers to have dementia by the age of 65.

Gluten is the protein found in wheat. Many people are either sensitive (gluten intolerant or have celiac disease) or allergic to gluten. Many people don't even know they are allergic to gluten and are often misdiagnosed with irritable bowel syndrome or another gastrointestinal disorder. It is believed that 83 percent of Americans who have celiac disease are undiagnosed or misdiagnosed with other conditions.[37] According to Dr. David Perlmutter, author of *Grain Brain*, eating foods that have high glycemic indexes, such as gluten, increases the chances of developing neurological disorders like Alzheimer's and dementia.[38] He notes that some people without celiac disease have neurological responses to gluten, including migraines and "brain fog." Gluten is found in rye, bulgur, couscous, semolina, barley, barley malt, triticale, einkorn, and kamut. Better choices for whole grains are rice, buckwheat, millet, quinoa, teff, amaranth, sorghum, and oats.

Sugar and sugar substitutes such as aspartame can act as toxins and cause chronic inflammation and upset hormone balance. It is also important to avoid processed foods because food-processing techniques such as extreme heating, irradiation, ionization, pasteurization, and sterilization may promote low-grade chronic inflammation by contributing to glycation (abnormal cross-linking of proteins) and oxidation of proteins and lipids. Certain at-home food preparations, such as frying, broiling, and grilling, act like food processing and increase glycation (as mentioned, AGEs).

A study conducted at University of California, Los Angeles (UCLA) in 2012 found that a diet high in fructose, another name for sugar, hinders learning and memory by slowing down the brain.[39] The study showed that rats that consumed high doses of fructose had damaged synaptic activity in the brain, and this impaired communication among brain cells. Heavy sugar intake caused the rats to develop a resistance to insulin, a hormone that controls blood sugar levels and also regulates the function of the brain cells. Insulin strengthens the synaptic connections between brain cells, helping them to communicate better and help form stronger memories. Basically, when the insulin levels in the brain are lowered as a result of excess sugar consumption, cognition can be impaired. Dr. Fernando Gomez-Pinilla, the lead author of the study and professor of neurosurgery at the David Geffen School of Medicine at UCLA, said, "Eating a high-fructose diet over long term alters your brain's ability to learn and remember information. Our findings illustrate that what you eat affects how you think."[40] He adds that consuming a diet high in omega-3 fatty acids to meals may help minimize the damage.

The problem is that the average American eats too much sugar! According to the United States Department of Agriculture, Americans consume roughly 47 pounds of cane sugar and 35 pounds of high-fructose corn syrup per year.[41] A sugar-heavy diet can increase the risk of developing Alzheimer's disease. The 2012 UCLA study found that insulin resistance and blood glucose levels (hallmarks of diabetes) are linked with greater risk of developing neurodegenerative disorders such as Alzheimer's.[42] The bottom line is it's best to avoid eating sugar, high-fructose corn syrup, and any processed, inexpensive liquid sweeteners and artificial sweeteners.

Fresh fruit is the best sweet-tooth satisfier for the brain. However, sometimes it's more fun to have a cookie, muffins, or piece of pie. In

The Memory Diet we created desserts that make eating sweets healthy and tasty. It's not about deprivation; it's about preservation.

We want to preserve our memory while still satisfying our sweet-tooth cravings. We created sweet treats that are made with pure organic fruit, raw honey, coconut sugar, and pure maple syrup. Honey is loaded with antioxidants that may help prevent cellular damage and memory loss. Honey helps the body absorb calcium, and calcium helps to aid brain health. The brain needs calcium to process thought and make decisions. Raw honey has polyphenols that enhances the memory.

Pure coconut sugar is harvested naturally from the coconut tree. It is found in the sap of the flowers of the coconut tree and has a low glycemic index, which translates into it being a healthier alternative to cane sugar, which has a high glycemic index. The glycemic index is a measurement of how a food affects the glucose levels in our body. A higher score means the greater our blood sugar will rise when we consume that food.

Coconut sugar contains glutamine and inositol, both of which help keep the heart and brain healthy. Pure maple syrup is an excellent source of manganese, which plays an important role in energy production and antioxidant defenses, and is necessary for normal brain and nerve function.

The recipes in Chapter 4 focus on clean eating and stay clear of processed foods that can damage the brain. Many processed foods contain too much salt. High sodium (salt) intake is associated with high blood pressure and other cardiovascular problems. Once again, if something is bad for the heart, then it's bad for the brain. A Mediterranean diet uses many spices and herbs instead of salt to enhance the flavors of foods. If you do eat processed food now and then, then try to avoid anything that has more than 500 mg. of sodium (salt) per serving.

Eating red meat is not good for you. It's high in saturated fats and is unhealthy for the heart. Eating red meat is also believed to contribute to Alzheimer's due to the fat that it is high in iron. A study from UCLA, suggests that iron accumulation on the brain is a contributing factor to Alzheimer's disease.[43] Using a special MRI technique, researchers found that iron had begun to accumulate in the brains of Alzheimer's patients.

Smoking is toxic to the body! Smoking increases the odds of getting dementia for those over 65 by nearly 80 percent and almost half of the people with mental illness are smokers.[44] Studies show that smokers don't remember people's name and faces as well as non-smokers do.[45] No one knows whether smoking directly impairs memory or is merely associated with memory loss because it causes illnesses that contribute memory loss. Smoking is especially common among people who are depressed, and depression weakens the memory. In addition, smoking increases the risk for stroke and hypertension, two other causes of memory impairment. Smoking can interfere with memory loss because it damages the lungs and constricts blood vessels to the brain, depriving it of oxygen and possibly harming neurons.

Maintaining a healthful lifestyle helps you to preserve your memory and slow cognitive decline, and it may even help you get back what you have lost. Making a commitment to your health will show results within time. You can keep your mind sharp, no matter what age you are.

CHAPTER 2

Foods for Thought: The Power of Diet

Your diet can influence not only the health of your body, but the health of your brain as well. The standard American diet is responsible for many serious health problems because it is filled with processed foods, sugars, simple carbohydrates, and saturated and trans fat. Eating a well-balanced diet that emphasizes certain foods can truly help your brain and form a protective barrier around what we value most: a lifetime of memories, acquired knowledge, and earned wisdom!

New research published by Martha Clare Morris, ScD, from Rush University Medical Center, shows a plant-based diet reduces the risk of Alzheimer's disease by 35 percent to 50 percent, depending on how diligently it's followed.[1] This new approach, formally called the Mediterranean Intervention Neurodegenerative Delay (MIND) diet, is a hybrid of the Mediterranean Diet and the Dietary Approaches to Stop Hypertension (DASH). This diet is associated with slower cognitive decline and is also great for the heart. Evidence shows that foods that are good for the heart are good for the brain. Your brain is nourished by one of your body's richest networks of blood vessels. Every heartbeat pumps about 20 to 25 percent of your blood to your head, where brain cells use at least 20 percent of the food and oxygen your blood carries.

The MIND diet is not the only research to support the fact that a Mediterranean diet can reduce your risk of dementia. In the July 2015 issue of the *Journal of the American Medical Association (JAMA)*, research was done on 447 men and women who were approximately 67 years in age. All patients had a series of dementia screens called neuropsychological test battery. No patients had evidence of dementia when they started the study. They found that memory was preserved and slightly improved in people on Mediterranean diets who used olive oil and ate nuts compared with people who simply lowered their dietary fat. In fact, in the non-Mediterranean diet group memory function actually declined by 17 percent.[2]

The MIND diet consists of leafy greens, vegetables, berries, nuts, beans, and whole grains as daily dietary staples. It also suggests eating fish and chicken in a very limited way. It suggests not consuming red meat, butter, margarine, cheese, sweets, pastries, and fried or fast food. These foods to avoid can more than double your risk of cognitive decline. To keep it simple, think in terms of the nutrition rainbow and aim to eat seven to eight colors from plant-based sources each day.

Plant-based foods are not only low in calories, but rich in nutrients that are an integral part to maintaining brain health. They include antioxidants (special vitamins and minerals) that help fight against inflammation and free radical damage in your nervous system. Following a plant-based diet that is rich in nuts, whole grains, extra-virgin olive oil (as well as coconut and avocado oil), and an abundance of fresh produce is beneficial to the brain.

The tasty recipes in this book are plant-based, dairy-free, gluten-free, and sugar-free. Gluten, a protein found in wheat, rye, and barley, can have severe effects on the gut as well as the brain. Many cases of neurological illness, known as gluten-sensitive idiopathic neuropathy, can be caused or exacerbated by gluten consumption. Dr. David Perlmutter, author of *Grain Brain*, claims eating foods with high glycemic indexes, which happen to be some of the most gluten-rich foods, increases the chances of developing neurological disorders like Alzheimer's and dementia.[3] Diets rich in gluten and dairy not only can contribute to celiac disease but can also cause neurological responses, which include migraines and "brain fog."

Dr. Perlmutter's research states the two main culprits contributing to Alzheimer's are excessive sugar and gluten consumption. It's becoming increasingly clear that the same pathological process that leads to insulin resistance and type 2 diabetes may also hold true for your brain. If you over-indulge on sugar and gluten, your brain becomes overwhelmed by the consistently high levels of glucose and insulin that blunt its insulin signaling, leading to impairments in your thinking and memory abilities that can eventually cause permanent brain damage.

Furthermore, when your liver is busy processing fructose (which your liver turns into fat), it severely hampers its ability to make cholesterol, an essential building block of your brain that is crucial for optimal brain function. Mounting evidence supports the notion that significantly reducing fructose consumption is a very important step for preventing Alzheimer's disease.

Preparing foods that are fresh, local, and organic are the ideal fuel foods for the brain. It is important to avoid processed foods because these foods are not digested well by the body. Cooking foods can be tricky because most foods that are cooked lose important digestive enzymes. For example, often people think that unsweetened jelly or concentrated apple juice is healthy to use, but in reality these are processed foods that are heated and reduced to a highly concentrated forms of sugar with all the enzymes and vitamins destroyed by the heating process. Plus, these processed foods are void of fiber! Processed foods turn into glucose that can easily turn into fat and create many health problems, including memory loss.

A study completed by Icahn School of Medicine at Mount Sinai Hospital showed that a diet high in glycotoxins called advanced glycation end products (AGEs), which are found in high concentration in well-done meat, is a risk factor in developing age-related dementia.[4] AGEs naturally form inside the body when proteins or fats combine with sugars (glycation). This affects the normal function of cells, making them more susceptible to damage and premature aging. AGEs are greater in animal-derived foods that are high in fat and protein, such as meats (especially red meats), which are prone to AGE formation through cooking. In contrast, carbohydrate-rich foods such as vegetables, fruits, and whole grains contain relatively few AGEs, even after cooking. Sugary foods and highly processed and prepackaged products also are high in AGEs.

Cooking methods that use high temperatures to brown or char foods, such as grilling, roasting, and broiling have the highest impact on the amount of AGEs consumed. The formation of new AGEs during cooking was prevented by the AGE inhibitory compound aminoguanidine and significantly reduced by cooking with moist heat, like steaming, using shorter cooking times, and cooking at lower temperatures. It's best to eat a plant-based diet for the brain; however, if one does cook animal products, cooking them with acidic ingredients such as lemon juice or vinegar reduces the AGEs.

The body naturally rids itself of harmful AGE compounds, but it has trouble eliminating them when too many are ingested through food. Basically, all the cells of the body cells are affected by the accumulation of AGEs. AGEs are linked to aging and also the development of worsening of many chronic illnesses, such as cardiovascular, liver, and Alzheimer's disease.

To reduce the damaging effects of AGEs on the brain:

» Limit grilling, broiling, frying, and microwaving foods. Substitute plant sources for protein instead of meat sources.
» Reduce the cooking temperature for baking to 250 degrees Fahrenheit.
» Cut down on processed foods. Many prepared foods have been exposed to high cooking temperatures to lengthen their shelf life. This process causes a higher AGE content in the foods.
» Eat an abundance of fresh fruits and vegetables. Both are excellent for the brain! Cooked or raw, they are naturally low in AGEs, and many contain compounds such as antioxidants that can decrease some of the damage done by AGEs. Vegetables and fruits contain dietary phytonutrients, which are found in the pigments of various colorful fruits and vegetables. One type of phytonutrient in particular—iridoids, which are found in deeply colored fruits such as blueberries—can lower AGEs in the body.

7 Brain-Boosting Food Groups

These are the seven "brain-boosting food groups" that the recipes in this book focus on.

1. Cruciferous Vegetables and Cabbage

Broccoli, cauliflower, bok choy, Brussels sprouts, cabbage, and kale contain folate and have carotenoids that lower homo-cysteine (amino acid) linked with cognitive impairment. Broccoli is one of the most popular vegetables in the United States. It is a super food for the whole body. It is rich in calcium, vitamin C, B vitamins, beta-carotene, iron, fiber, and vitamin K. These nutrients protect against free radicals, keep blood flowing well, and remove heavy metals that can damage the brain. These vegetables contain lignans, which have been shown to benefit assorted brain functions, such as thinking, reasoning, remembering, imagining, and learning new words. Cruciferous vegetables are also high in glucosinolates, which help promote levels of acetylcholine, a vital neurotransmitter in the central nervous system.

Red cabbage is full of polyphenols, a powerful antioxidant that benefits the brain and heart. Red cabbage also has glucosinolates compounds that fight cancer.

2. Leafy Greens

Spinach, collard greens, mustard greens, turnip greens, romaine lettuce, and red leaf lettuce are all foods that are high in folic acid (folate, also known as vitamin B9). Folate improves cognition function and helps reduce the risk of Alzheimer's disease.

Spinach can prevent or delay dementia. The nutrients in spinach prevent damage to DNA, cancer cell growth, and tumor growth, as well as slow the effects of aging on the brain. Spinach is also a good source of folate and vitamin E.

3. Seeds and Nuts

Seeds and nuts are high in omega-3 fatty acids that may help prevent Alzheimer's decease and dementia. People whose diets contain daily omega-3s have 26 percent less risk of having brain lesions that cause dementia compared to those who did not.[5] Omega-3s provide many benefits, including improving learning and helping to fight against such mental disorders as depression and mood disorders and schizophrenia.

Many people eat cold-water fish to get their omega-3s. Yet eating fish is not necessary. In fact, due to our polluted waters, fish has way too much mercury and is not the best choice for omega-3s. You can get the essential fatty acids (EPAs), and docosahexaenoic acid (DHA), and docosapentaenoic acid (DPA) found in omega-3s from vegetarian sources such as walnuts, flaxseeds, and chia seeds. Flaxseed provides alpha linolenic acid, which converts into DHA and DPA omega-3s in the body.

Chia seeds are rich in omega-3 fatty acids and both soluble and insoluble fiber. These powerful little seeds help control blood glucose levels, are anti-inflammatory, aid in hydration, and also contain many antioxidants. Sunflower seeds and other seeds, like pumpkin, contain a rich mix of protein, omega fatty acids, zinc, choline, vitamin E, and B vitamins. These seeds contain tryptophan, which the brain converts into serotonin to boost mood and combat depression.

Walnuts and almonds are extremely good for the brain and nervous system. They are great sources of omega-3 and omega-6 fatty acids, vitamin B6, and vitamin E. Vitamin E has been shown to prevent many forms of dementia by protecting the brain from free radicals, and it improves brain power. Cashews, hazelnuts, pecans, peanuts (technically a legume), and pistachios all contain omega-3s and omega-6s, vitamin E, folate, vitamin B6, and magnesium.

4. Fruits, Grapes, and Berries

The brain is highly susceptible to oxidative damage. Fruits contain anthocyanin that protects the brain from further damage caused by free radicals. They also have anti-inflammatory properties and contain antioxidants and vitamins C and E.

Fruits such as tomatoes and cucumbers are great brain foods. Tomatoes contain lycopene, a very powerful antioxidant that combats dementia and may also improve mood balance. Most people consider a cucumber a vegetable, yet it's actually related to the melon family. The anti-inflammatory flavonol and fisetin in cucumber play an important role in brain health. Fisetin protects against progressive memory loss and cognitive decline.

Avocados are also an excellent fruit for the brain. Avocados are loaded with antioxidants including vitamin E, which protects the body and brain from free radical damage. They are also a good source of potassium and vitamin K, which protects the brain from the risk of stroke. Avocados are smooth and creamy because of their fat content. They are rich in a fatty acid called oleic acid, which helps to build the coating of insulation, known as myelin (found in white matter of the brain). Myelin helps information travel at speeds of up to 200 miles per hour. Neurons without myelin (gray matter) process information at slower speeds.

Pumpkins and squash are fruits that contain vitamin A, folate, and iron that help with cognition. Folate is effective in preventing cognitive decline and dementia during aging.

Red and black grapes contain resveratrol, a powerful antioxidant that helps prevent dementia. A study done on mice and published in *The FASEB Journal* revealed that red wine might stop the formation of brain proteins tied to Alzheimer's disease because it contains resveratrol.[6] You can get resveratrol from eating organic red or black grapes, or drinking grape juice. Drinking lots of wine will not stop the development of Alzheimer's disease and can actually increase one's chances of getting dementia.[7]

Blueberries contain flavonoids, compounds that are thought to enhance memory. Flavonoids have been shown to enhance spatial memory in both animals and humans, and fruit-derived flavonoids are thought to be especially potent, making blueberries a perfect choice. Other dark berries are good for the brain too, like blackberry, açai, and goji berries.

5. Beans, Legumes, and Whole Grains

Beans and legumes are excellent sources of complex carbohydrates. These complex carbohydrates are also mixed with fiber that slows absorption, giving us a steady supply of glucose for the brain without the risks of sugar spikes associated with many other sugar sources. Beans and legumes are also rich in folic acid, a B vitamin critical to brain function and essential omega fatty acids. They also have iron, magnesium, potassium, and choline, a B vitamin that boosts acetylcholine (a neurotransmitter critical for brain function).

Like beans and legumes, whole grains are rich in complex carbohydrates, fiber, and some omega-3 fatty acids that shield the heart and brain from damaging sugar spikes, cholesterol, blood clots, and more.

Grains also contain B vitamins that have an effect on blood flow to the brain. Whole grains such as quinoa (used as a grain but truly a seed) and oats are an excellent source of complex carbohydrates and fiber that balance blood sugar while providing the essential glucose the brain craves. Gluten-free, protein-rich quinoa is also a good source for iron (to keep the blood oxygenated) and B vitamins (to balance mood and protect blood vessels). Oats contain omega-3 fatty acids, folate, and potassium. This fiber-rich super food can lower levels of LDL (or bad) cholesterol and help keep arteries clear. It's a heart-friendly food, which in turn is a brain-friendly food.

6. Olive, Coconut, Macadamia, and Avocado Oils

Extra-virgin olive oil contains a type of natural phenolic compound called oleocanthal that has antioxidant and anti-inflammatory properties. According to a study published in *ACS Chemical Neuroscience*, research done on mice suggests that oleocanthal helps shuttle abnormal Alzheimer's disease proteins out of the brain.[8] Coconut oil has shown to help the brain as well. Coconut oil is a rich source of medium-chain triglycerides (MCTs), which are broken down into ketones. Higher ketone values (derivatives from fat that are the only other fuel source aside from glucose for the brain to function) have been associated with greater improvement in Alzheimer's patients. The MCTs in coconut oil may provide therapeutic benefits for memory-impaired adults. Coconut oil may help boost energy levels and endurance, as it is not stored in the body like other fats and breaks down much quicker in the liver, and is used like a carbohydrate. Macadamia oil actually has a higher level of monounsaturated fats than olive oil. It contains oleic acid, the same type of fat in avocados that can help lower triglyceride levels. Macadamia oil has the ideal balance of omega-3 and omega-6 fats—healthy fats for the brain. Avocado oil also contains high quantities of monounsaturated fatty acids. A study published in the October 2012 issue of the Federation of American Societies for Experimental Biology found that monounsaturated fatty acids helped protect nerve cells in the brain known as astrocytes, which provide support to information carrying nerves.[9] In the laboratory animal study, monounsaturated fats improved the ability of the brain to control muscles in animals with impaired astrocyte function. Fish oil, also tested in this study, did not provide the same benefits. Researchers concluded that monounsaturated fats may be helpful in the treatment of certain brain disorders.

7. Brain Spices

Turmeric is a staple spice in Asian and Indian cuisines and is best known as part of curry powder. Curcumin is a plant chemical found in turmeric. It inhibits a neurotoxin that has been linked to neurodegenerative disorders and shows promise as both an antioxidation and anti-inflammatory agent.

Black pepper is the most widely used spice on the planet and it contains piperine. Piperine can help inhibit the breakdown of dopamine and serotonin (two neurotransmitters crucial to brain health and mood regulation). It also appears to help control the flow of calcium in the brain which gives anti-seizure effects.

Garlic helps thin the blood, which increases the flow throughout the body, including to the brain. It also helps battle free radical damage to the brain, which has been associated with degenerative conditions like Alzheimer's. Garlic has been shown to be effective in preventing and battling tumors in the brain, too.

Ginger is a powerful antioxidant that has anti-inflammatory properties and significantly improves cognitive function. In a study published by Evidence-Based Complementary and Alternative Medicine, women between the ages of 50 and 60 in Thailand were given cognitive function and memory assessments prior to taking ginger supplements for two months. Half the women were given ginger supplements and the other half of women were given a placebo. The women who took ginger supplements showed "a significant improvement in cognitive functions and an enhanced working memory compared to women who were given a placebo."[10] The researchers reports concluded that ginger extract enhanced the women's attention and cognitive processing capabilities.

Cinnamon boosts the activity of the brain by removing nervous tension and diminishing memory loss. Smelling cinnamon may boost cognitive function and memory performance of certain tasks, and increase one's alertness and concentration.

Rosemary has been shown to improve memory and cognitive function with its scent alone. It improves blood flow to the brain and improves mood. It is a powerful detoxifier that can help fight cancer, boosts energy, and combats aging in the skin.

Sage is a wonderful herb that has anti-inflammatory and powerful memory-enhancing qualities. In trials, even small amounts of sage have been shown to significantly boost memory recall. The root of the Chinese sage contains compounds that are very similar to the drugs used to treat Alzheimer's disease. The herb has been used for more than 1,000 years to treat brain-related problems. Sage has been found to improve the interconnectivity of the different parts of the brain. Carnosic acid, an antioxidant found in sage can even cross the blood barrier to halt free radical damage in the brain. The same antioxidant increases our own production of glutathione, an important anti-aging, antioxidant, which improves circulation to the brain by dilating the cerebral middle arteries. Glutathione is actually used to treat all sorts of brain diseases, from autism to Alzheimer's. Having good blood flow to the brain is vital.

Green tea is loaded with antioxidants! Matcha Tea, derived from green tea, has even a higher level of antioxidants as well as a higher content of chlorophyll. Both extracts enhance cognitive function, especially the working memory of the brain.

All these spices and herbs help protect the brain and reduce inflammation. Incorporating these seven brain-boosting foods into your diet will help decrease your risk of memory loss and other illnesses. The delicious dishes in Chapter 4 are filled with foods that are not only great for the brain but for the entire body!

CHAPTER 3

Stocking a Mindful Kitchen

It's a good idea to keep a variety of kitchen staples on hand. Having the right kitchen supplies—supplies that are "brain friendly"—makes it easy to prepare healthy meals and snacks including the recipes in this book. It is important to use whole foods and whole-food products that are unprocessed (or minimally processed) so they are close to their natural, nutrient-packed state. This means whole foods, including fresh fruits and vegetables, whole grains, and beans that preferably are locally grown. It also means using unrefined natural sweeteners like fruit juice, date sugar, coconut sugar, raw honey, or maple syrup. Ideally you use organically grown foods, because not only are they better for you, they are better for the environment.

Why Organic?

Organic foods are grown in rich soil that is free of pesticides and synthetic fertilizers. They do not contain chemical additives, hormones, or preservatives. And because they are very close to their natural state, they usually taste better. Many pesticides contain neurotoxins that are designed to damage the nervous system of insects. Studies in the environmental health department at Harvard University in Southern Denmark show that pesticides designed to harm the nervous system of insects may be harmful to the human brain.[1]

Another important reason to choose organic is to avoid genetically modified (GM) food, which comes from genetically modified organisms (GMOs). Simply put, the genes of GM plants have been altered or artificially manipulated to mix and match the DNA of totally different species, often for the purpose of growing a bigger, better version of the crop or to create one that is resistant to pesticides and herbicides. The increase in pesticides and chemicals on our foods and in our environment is disrupting the natural healthy bacteria in our stomachs and throwing everything out of whack, which could be adding to an increase in food allergies as well as having a negative impact on the brain function!

Nearly 80 percent of the corn and more than 90 percent of the soybeans grown in the United States are genetically modified.[2] The most popular herbicide-resistant GM crops are Monsanto company's Roundup Ready crops, which are engineered to be resistant to Monsanto's own broad spectrum herbicide, Roundup, which contains the herbicide glyphosate. Because the plants are resistant to the herbicide, growers are able to douse their fields with it, killing the weeds and pests without harming the crops themselves. Growers no longer need to till the soil to control weeds. Though there have been many arguments in favor of genetically modified foods, there are a growing number of reasons against them.

Science has discovered that almost 90 percent of the serotonin in the body is produced in the digestive process.[3] More than 30 neurotransmitters (brain chemicals) are created by the digestive process and the bacteria found in your gut. GMOs and glyphosate have a damaging effect on digestive bacteria.[4] Poor digestion creates a multitude of physical and emotional problems. Poor digestion can lead to poor "gut health," which is often the culprit for autism and depression.[5] Glyphosate harms gut bacteria, which in turn affects brain health. Glyphosate also disrupts the ability of the liver to detoxify and this allows toxins to enter the body and cross the blood brain barrier and further intrude on brain health.

9 Is Fine

Another way to avoid genetically modified produce is by checking the price look-up (PLU) code, which is found on a tiny label that is stuck on the fruit or vegetable. The PLU code for GM produce has five numbers that begin with the number 8. Organically grown fruits and vegetables have five numbers that begin with the number 9. The PLU code for non-GMO produce that is grown through conventional farming methods (which likely means the use of pesticides, herbicides, and/or chemical fertilizers) has only four numbers. An easy way to remember is organic varieties is by keeping in mind that "9 is fine."

Where to Shop

Fortunately, due to an increasing demand for whole and organic foods, when it comes to shopping, you have a number of good options. Farmers' markets that sell fresh organic produce are located in towns and cities throughout the United States. Local farmers sell freshly picked fruits and vegetables that increase the nutritional value of the produce. As soon as that apple is picked, its vitamin and mineral content begins to diminish. Most of the produce found on supermarket shelves was picked four to seven days earlier and transported an average of 1,500 miles. Local farmers' markets assure fresher foods than what you'll find in the supermarket, and you will be supporting local growers. (To locate farmers' markets in your area, visit *www.ams.usda.gov/farmersmarkets/map.htm*.)

Natural foods markets also sell whole foods like fruits, vegetables, whole grains, and whole-grain products that are typically organic. Many of the larger stores offer extensive selections, and their product turnover rate is usually quick, which is a good indication of freshness. Although natural foods markets are often more expensive than other stores, they tend to support local farmers and sustainable agriculture practices. Sustainable agriculture is a way of growing or raising food, including animals, in an ecologically and ethically responsible way using practices that protect the environment, safeguard human health, are humane to farm animals, and provide fair treatment to workers. Eating sustainably follows these principles. We encourage sustainable agriculture because it provides numerous health benefits, including less exposure to harmful substances such as pesticides, antibiotic-resistant bacteria, and unhealthful food additives. Foods that are sustainable usually have higher nutrients and antioxidants, too. We like to eat sustainably because we know that we are also supporting a more environmentally and socially responsible food system!

Many supermarkets are beginning to carry whole foods and organic products. They are conveniently located, which is a plus; however, the selection is often limited and product turnover may be slow, which means compromised freshness.

Finally, you can also purchase organic foods online. Another thing to keep in mind when buying organic is that packaged foods often contain multiple ingredients. The word *organic* appearing on a label does not necessarily mean that the product is 100-percent organic. Organic product labeling can be confusing. It is important to note that even if a producer is certified organic, using the USDA organic seal is voluntary. In addition, the process of becoming certified is very demanding and costly, and not all organic producers are willing to go through that.

Be Aware of Kitchenware

It is imperative to be aware of pesticides on produce, the mercury in fish, the chemicals in our food, the products we clean with, and the products we use on our bodies—and to also realize the importance of the kitchenware you use. Kitchenware can make a difference in your overall health, too! Kitchenware can contain chemicals such as aluminum, lead, copper, mercury, and plastic that can leach into your food. Avoid aluminum cookware. Aluminum is a metal found in food additives, car exhaust, tobacco smoke, foil cans, ceramics, antacids, antidiarrheal medications, and infant immunizations. Prolonged or intensive exposure to aluminum has been shown in some studies to be associated with nerve damage and formation of amyloid plaques in the brain.[6] Amyloid plaques themselves are associated with the development of Alzheimer's disease and other forms of dementia that interfere with your basic cognitive function.[7] Nonstick pans, pots, bakeware, and utensils using Teflon may be convenient, but they are made from perfluorinated compounds, which have been linked to cancer and reproductive problems. Ceramic dishware can crack and chip because the glazes used in ceramic dishware often contain lead, which can leach into foods. Even dish racks made of plastic-coated wire should be substituted with stainless steel dish racks. It's best to use glass bakeware, and stainless steel or cast iron pots and pans, as well as stainless steel and glass mixing bowls. Although heavy metal poisoning is rare, its effects on the brain and nervous system can be extensive and it can lead to cognitive decline and memory loss.

Some handy cooking utensils in the our kitchen are a cooking timer, set of measuring cups and spoons, a 1 1/2-inch ice cream scoop (great to scoop out cookie dough onto a baking sheet or fill muffin liners with batter), a rubber end spatula (ideal for scraping the last bit of a mixture around a bowl), and an immersion blender.

Mindful Kitchen Must-Haves

We have put together a list of products we recommend to keep handy in your kitchen. When buying packaged items, always check ingredients labels and carefully—even products you have bought before, as manufacturers often change product ingredients without warning. Understanding organic labeling can be a little confusing, especially for products that contain more than one ingredient. In an effort to help consumers understand the organic content of the food they buy, the USDA has established the following labeling rules:

Single-Ingredient Foods: For fruits, vegetables, and other single-ingredient foods, a sticker version of the USDA Organic seal may appear on the products themselves or on a sign near them.

Multi-Ingredient Foods: For packaged foods that contain more than one ingredient, the following labeling terms are used to indicate their organic content: If the label says **100% Organic** it must contain 100-percent organic ingredients. It is permitted to use the USDA seal. If the label says **Organic,** then the product must contain 95- to 100-percent organic ingredients. It is permitted to use the USDA seal. If the label says **Made With Organic Ingredients,** the product must contain at least 70 percent organic ingredients. If the product says **Contains Organic Ingredients,** then it has less than 70 percent organic ingredients.

It is also important to know that even if a producer is certified organic, using the USDA Organic seal is voluntary. In addition, the process of becoming certified is very demanding, and not all producers of organic foods are willing to go through it, especially small farming operations. For this reason, never hesitate to ask vendors, such as your local farmers' markets, how their products are grown. Many growers may not be certified organic but instead claim their produce is "pesticide-free," which is still good.

Milk Substitutes

Rice milk (light and mild flavor, and easily accessible), oat milk (mild flavor), coconut milk (thick and rich flavor), almond milk (naturally sweet), hazelnut milk (mildly sweet), quinoa milk (light and mild), flaxseed milk (flaxmilk) and hemp milk (has a rich, nutty flavor). For optimal nutrition, choose organic varieties that are fortified with calcium, and vitamins D, B, and E.

Dairy-free buttermilk: Mix 1 tablespoon lemon juice or apple cider vinegar with 1 cup of milks listed above. Let sit a few minutes to thicken.

Dairy-free cream: When a recipe should call for a dairy-free cream, you can use the same amount of potato puree instead.

Butter Substitutes

Butter gives a rich flavor, and in cookies extra-virgin olive oil can be substituted as well as sesame seed oil, safflower oil, and sunflower seed oil. Unrefined coconut oil (which is solid at room temperature) can add the thickness that butter would. There are vegan butter substitutes, such as the brand Earth Balance, which has no trans fats and creates the buttery taste so many holiday cookies require.

Cream Substitutes

Cream creates a smooth and sometimes-fluffy texture in baked goods. It adds richness and can make for a satin-like quality. The richness of coconut milk can be a good replacement for cream. Another good homemade replacement is to blend one part cashews and one part water until smooth.

Egg Substitutes

Ener-G Egg Replacer is an egg-replacement product available at the grocery store. However, we prefer to use any of the following as a substitute for eggs. To make your own egg-free substitute for baking purposes, try any of the following ingredient combinations, each of which is equivalent to one egg:

1 T. flaxseed meal or chia seeds + 3 T. warm water (Let sit 3 minutes.)
1 T. agar flakes dissolved in 1/4 c. hot water then blended until smooth
1 tsp. baking powder + 1 T. apple cider vinegar
1 T. agar plus 1 T. water
1/4 c. mashed potatoes
1/2 tsp. baking powder + 3 T. applesauce

Oils

Not all oils are created equal. Keep these basic categories in mind when cooking:

For baking: Coconut or a high oleic safflower or sunflower oil works best.

For quick stir-frying: Use coconut, macadamia, or avocado oil. These oils stand up to heat best. You never want to over heat oil where you see smoke coming up, as this causes the oil to oxidize. If the oil smokes, discard it; this signals that the oil has been damaged.

For quick sautéing: Use coconut, olive, macadamia, avocado, sesame, or high oleic safflower or sunflower oil. We use extra-virgin olive oil, as it has heart- and brain-healthy monounsaturated fats and phenols that have protective compounds that provide numerous benefits. But to maximize the health benefits, we recommend using it raw for salads and dips, and for lower-heat cooking. Refined oils recommended for high-heat cooking and deep-frying are labeled as "high oleic," as in the safflower and sunflower oils. We do not recommend any deep frying or "browning" foods because the high AGEs are not healthy for the brain.

For dipping, dressings, and marinades: Use olive, flax, toasted sesame, macadamia, or walnut oil. These oils have terrific flavor that makes them ideal for dipping and dressings.

We do not use canola oil because more than 90 percent of canola grown in the United States is GMO. Soy, corn, canola, and cotton are the most common genetically engineered (GE) crops.

Canola oil is bred from rapeseed. Many years ago the rapeseed contained high levels of erucic acid considered harmful to humans. Today's canola oil goes through a very harsh process and contains less than 2 percent of this controversial fatty acid. Mass-market oils generally are extracted with toxic solvents such as hexane and undergo harsh treatments to remove the solvent, and more chemicals, high heat, and straining are used to deodorize and bleach the oils, creating inferior oil.

We use oils that have been mechanically pressed from the seed without using chemical solvents. These oils are known as "expeller pressed." When it comes to olive, avocado, and walnut oils we purchase "cold-pressed," which only needs expeller pressing and centrifuging to be made.

We recommend storing oils in an airtight glass bottle in a cool, dark place. For oils that will sit unused for longer than one month, storing in the refrigerator is ideal. Air, heat, and light cause oils to oxidize and turn rancid. Coconut oil tends to be solid at room temperature. To get it to a liquid state, place it in a pan and cook it over a low heat.

Natural oils should smell and taste fresh and pleasant.

Note: Applesauce works as a wonderful binding agent and is also a great substitute for eggs, oil, or shortening when you want to reduce the fat. One-half cup unsweetened applesauce is equivalent to one egg.

Beans

Studies have shown that people who eat more legumes have a lower risk of heart disease, and the phytochemicals found in beans protect the brain, too![8] Beans contain a wide range of cancer-fighting plant chemicals, specifically isoflavones and phytosterols, which are associated with reduced cancer risk. Another bonus is that beans are high in soluble fiber, which plays an important role in controlling blood cholesterol levels. Beans contain saponins and phytosterols, which help lower cholesterol and help the brain also. There are some beans, such as soybeans, that contain substances that may interfere with the absorption of beta-carotene and vitamins B12 and D. It's important to slowly cook beans because cooked beans make vitamin absorption easier.

Dry beans keep up to a year in an airtight container in a cool, dry environment away from direct sunlight.

To cook beans: Soak dry beans in cold water about eight hours or overnight. Soaking the beans helps hydrate the beans and considerably shortens the cooking time. It's best to soak beans in a cool place or refrigerator to avoid any fermentation. Always wash beans thoroughly before soaking.

Add one or two bay leaves to a pot of beans to bring out the flavor of the beans. Discard the bay leaves after the beans have cooked. Other flavor enhancers you can put in the pot of the beans and then discard afterward are peppercorns and a whole peeled yellow onion.

Add any seasonings, herbs, or spices toward the end of the cooking process, because their cooking process tends to diminish the longer they cook. To reduce cooking time up to 10 minutes try adding acidic ingredients such as lemon juice and vinegar.

Black beans: Also known as turtle beans. Rich in magnesium, they have a velvety texture and subtly sweet taste. Great in Mexican dishes and veggie burgers.

Black-eyed peas: Small, plump, and spotted beans. An excellent source of folate. Have an earthy taste.

Borlotti beans: Creamy texture with an earthy flavor. Known as cranberry beans because of their deep red spots. Great in Italian dishes.

Cannellini beans: Large, rosy-beige beans also known as white Italian kidney beans. Have a delicate flavor. A versatile bean that can be combined in pasta and salads or blended for dips.

Chickpeas, or garbanzo beans: The most consumed beans in the world! Round and firm with a nutty flavor. The basis for hummus, a tasty dip and spread!

Fava beans: Emerald green when fresh, with a firm texture and subtle nutty flavor. Great in salads.

Great Northern beans: Small, white, kidney-shaped beans that are high in calcium. Good in salads.

Kidney beans: Known for its reddish skin and white interior. Packed with protein and brain-healthy nutrients such as omega-3 fatty acids and iron. Great in stews, soups, and chili, and on salads.

Lentils: Tiny beans that are tender and savory. Because these beans are small they do not require soaking. Wonderful in soups, salads, and veggie burgers.

Lima beans: Green, flat, oval-shaped beans that have a buttery flavor. Their starchy interior can turn mushy, so it's best to steam these beans.

Pinto beans: Light brown beans that are high in fiber and protein. Have an earthy, smooth flavor. Excellent in Mexican dishes and veggie burgers.

A note about soy: Soybeans are high in fiber and protein, but unfortunately, more than 90 percent of the soybeans in the United States are genetically modified. Always get organic soy products. The vast majority of soy consumed in the United States is highly processed. The soybeans are cracked, hulled, crushed, or subjected to solvent extraction to separate their oils from the rest of the bean. What is left behind after oil extraction is defatted soy flour that's then further processed to produce a protein concentrate called protein isolate that isn't worth consuming. A better soy protein choice is organic tempeh. Tempeh is a form of soy that is closer to soy in its whole food form and is fermented. Fermentation increases the digestibility of soy (especially its proteins) and increases nutrient absorption

Flours

Oat (gluten-free), brown rice, sorghum, amaranth, buckwheat, chickpea (garbanzo), millet, potato, lentil, chestnut, corn, tapioca, Montina, flax, teff, almond, and quinoa

Most of the time these flours can't be substituted equally for wheat flour, and they require varying amounts of xantham gum (binding agent) from recipe to recipe.

Baking Products and Thickeners

Baking powder (aluminum-free and albumin-free), baking soda, arrowroot, tapioca flour, agar powder, potato starch

Make sure baking powder does not contain lecithin, which could be derived from soy or egg source. Xanthan gum brings a springiness to breads and is used to help hold flour together that could otherwise be crumbly.

Nuts and Seeds

Flaxseeds, flaxseed meal, pumpkin seeds, sesame seeds, chia seeds, sunflower butter, and tahini (sesame seed butter)

Please note if you are allergic to tree nuts, these seeds (with the exception of sesame seeds) are rarely allergic and considered acceptable. Be aware, however, that although sesame seeds are not on the current top allergens by the FDA reactions to them—often serious—are on the rise, and sesame seeds are often called the ninth top food allergen. (In our allergen-free cookbooks we address the top eight allergens and sometimes have people write us to include sesame seeds in this list.) Again, check the labels, because some seed butters are manufactured in facilities that also manufacture nut butters.

Almonds, brazil nuts, cashews, hazelnuts, macadamia nuts, pecans, peanuts (really a legume), pine nuts, pistachios, walnuts

The most common nut butters are peanut butter, almond butter, and cashew butter.

Note: Coconut is used in many of the recipes because coconut is good for the brain and is tasty. Coconut is not a nut, but coconut oil is excellent for the brain and a great oil to cook with. When we use coconut oil we use organic pure coconut oil. It can be solid at room temperature, and it's easier to measure when it's in a liquid state that can be done by slightly warming it up in a small pot. We use unsweetened shredded coconut in many recipes and you can use the reduced-fat version, which we have found to taste the same, in the recipes. All pure coconut sugar, unsweetened coconut water, cream, and water are also included in the recipes.

Breads and Bread Products

Gluten-free/allergen-free varieties of bread and bread crumbs, bagels, buns, muffins, pitas, and rolls; brown rice tortillas; corn tortillas

Please note that brown rice tortillas are good for quesadillas but they are not easy to wrap around for burrito-type fillings. They are very stiff in structure.

Cereals (dry, ready to eat)

Gluten-free/allergen-free varieties, such as amaranth flakes, corn flakes, flax flakes, oat cereals, quinoa cereals, buckwheat cereals, puffed millet, puffed corn, and puffed rice

Beware of cereals that are highly processed and filled with additives, preservatives, and sugar. We recommend making your own cereals, such as Cashew Coconut Granola (page 177) and Grain-Free Granola (page 182).

Fresh Fruits (preferably organic)

Some common fruits: apples, bananas, berries, peaches, pears, melons, and citrus fruits (lemons, oranges, grapefruits, tangerines, mandarins, and clementines)

There are rare cases where someone has an allergic reaction to fruits such as apples or cantaloupe. It's not necessarily something that is inherent in the fruit, but instead it's the birch pollen that's commonly found on the surface of raw apples that can cause an itchy throat. Eating melons such as cantaloupe can also cause an itchy throat because of ragweed pollen that surrounds the fruit.

Try to eat organic dried fruit that has no sulfur in it. Often people can get an allergic reaction to dried fruit from the preservative of sulfates, which is also found in wine, that may cause an itchy jaw or flushed face.

Fresh Vegetables (preferably organic)

Some common vegetables: avocados, broccoli, cabbage, carrots, cauliflower, corn (organic only), cucumbers, eggplant, garlic, lettuce, kale, mushrooms, onions, peas, potatoes, scallions, spinach, squash, sweet potatoes (or yams), tomatoes

Sweeteners (preferably organic)

Our primary recommendations for sweeteners are fresh fruit and unprocessed sweeteners such as raw honey, pure maple syrup, and organic coconut sugar. Date sugar tends to clump up and get hard, so you have to use it soon after opening it. Coconut sugar (this is unsweetened and made from coconut tree sap), fruit juice (orange, apple, pear), fruit concentrate (frozen), monk fruit, honey, stevia and pure maple syrup are all choices for sweeteners, in moderation.

Canned and Bottled Goods

Beans (black beans, chickpeas, kidney beans, etc.), corn (organic only), fruit-sweetened jams, olives, pumpkin puree, tomato sauce

Make sure the cans used are bisphenol A (BPA) free and bisphenol S (BPS) free. These chemicals found in plastics tend to leach into the body. Studies have shown that BPA and BPS have been linked to all sorts of health problems, including breast and prostate cancers, heart trouble, type 2 diabetes, autism, liver tumors, asthma, infertility, and proper brain development. The best way to protect yourself from BPA, BPS, and their chemical cousins is to avoid plastic whenever possible, including plastics that claim they are “BPA-free.” Replace plastic water bottles with high-quality stainless steel bottles. Look for glass food-storage containers and ditch plastic containers. Avoid canned food whenever possible. Some environmentally aware companies, such as Eden Foods, use only companies that use vegetable-based canned food linings. Also, wash your hands after throwing away store receipts. Most receipts have coating on the paper that contains BPA or BPS, and has been shown to easily seep into the skin. Better yet, opt for an e-mail of your receipts to avoid coated paper receipts.

Snack Foods and Frozen Desserts

Raisins and other dried fruit (unsulfured); allergen-free products free of gluten such as flax crackers, oat crackers, popcorn, rice cakes, and rice crackers; baked corn chips and unsweetened fruit rollups or strips; frozen items such as fruit sorbets and homemade fruit juice popsicles

Pasta and Noodles

Brown rice pasta, corn pasta, quinoa pasta, buckwheat noodles, papadini lentil/bean pasta, lentil pasta, rice noodles (rice sticks)

Seasonings and Flavor Enhancers

Apple cider vinegar, balsamic vinegar, black pepper, carob powder, cinnamon, fresh/dried herbs(basil, rosemary, thyme, cilantro, oregano), garlic powder, garlic salt, ketchup, lemons, limes, mustard, nutmeg, pickles, salsa, sea salt, Tabasco or other hot sauce, vanilla extract (wheat-free and gluten-free)

Grains and Flours

Amaranth flour, brown rice, brown rice flour, buckwheat flour, chickpeas(garbanzo beans), chickpea flour, cornmeal, millet, oats(gluten-free), oat flour(gluten-free), potato flour, quinoa, quinoa flour, tapioca flour, sorghum flour, and teff flour

Wheat flour (1 c.) used as an ingredient in baked goods, and as a thickener in soups and sauces: 3/4 c. brown rice flour, 3/4 c. potato flour, 3/4 c. chickpea flour, 1 c. tapioca flour, or 1 1/4 c. oat flour.

Suggested flour combinations: 2/3 c. brown rice flour + 1/4 c. potato flour + 2 T. tapioca flour.

White sugar (1 c.) used as an ingredient in baked goods, desserts, and smoothies: 3/4 c. date sugar, 3/4 c. honey, 3/4 c. maple syrup, 3/4 c. rice syrup.

Friend Fats

According to the American Heart Association, a heart-healthy diet can contain up to 30 percent of calories from fat, provided that most of the fat is unsaturated.[9] Unsaturated fats, which include monounsaturated and polyunsaturated varieties, are "friendly fats" that lower harmful LDL cholesterol levels. Monounsaturated fats are found in olive, macadamia, and coconut oils. Olive oil is well-known for its high content of heart-healthy monounsaturated fats. However, macadamia nut oil is composed primarily of omega-3 fatty acids, which research has found to be effective in the treatment and prevention of a variety of different conditions, including cardiovascular disease, stroke, and even Alzheimer's disease.[10] Macadamia oil is ideal for cooking at higher temperatures because it has a high smoke point. Polyunsaturated fats are found in avocado, corn, flax, grape seed, safflower, sesame, sunflower, and walnut oils.

Foe Fats

Saturated fats are not your friends! They increase LDL cholesterol (the bad cholesterol), which clogs arteries and can lead to heart disease. Saturated fat, found mainly in animal sources like whole milk, butter, and fatty meats, has also been linked to an increased risk of type-2 diabetes. Another "foe" to avoid is hydrogenated fat. This type of fat is created when hydrogen is added to an oil (often unsaturated) to make it solid at room temperature. During this process, the fat becomes more saturated. Trans fats, considered the worst of the saturated fats, are created during the processing of foods through partial hydrogenation. Trans fats are often found in commercial products such as crackers, chips, and baked goods, and frozen items like waffles and French fries.

Recipe Choices

The recipes in this book use heart- and brain-healthy fats. These fats are cold-pressed, extra-virgin olive oils and organic coconut oil. The beneficial essential fatty acids they contain are also critical for nerve and brain functioning. Unfortunately, as mentioned previously, many commercial varieties of these oils are subjected to chemical and heat processing that causes the formation of harmful free radicals. These harmful free radicals can be avoided by using organic, cold-pressed, minimally processed oils.

Be aware that oats and oat flour are often processed in facilities that also handle wheat (and other gluten-containing grains such as rye and barley), so cross-contamination may occur. Make sure to purchase varieties that are certified wheat free or gluten free. Having these ingredients stocked in the kitchen make cooking easy, fun, and brain healthy!

Fruit and Veggie Wash

Always wash your fruits and vegetables before eating. Even organic varieties are likely to contain bacteria from processing, shipping, and handling. Here's the simple recipe we use and recommend:

1. Place 1 c. water and 2 T. fresh lemon juice, vinegar, salt, or baking soda in a spray bottle, and shake well.
2. Spray fruit or veggies with the wash, scrub gently with your hands, and rinse with cold water.
3. Store any remaining wash in the refrigerator.

Even if you do not make a veggie rinse, still make sure you clean your vegetables and fruits well with cold water.

Some Helpful Tips

Here are some helpful, quick tips and guidelines before preparing the delicious recipes in Chapter 4:

- » If you choose to use honey, instead you can use equal amounts of maple syrup or coconut sugar. Sometimes honey crystallizes. If this happens, place it in a heat-resistant glass cup or container, and place it in a pan or bowl of hot water. As it begins to heat up, stir the honey until it returns to a smooth liquid state.
- » If a recipe calls for oil and a liquid sweetener, first measure the oil. After emptying out the oil, use the same measuring

cup (don't clean it) to measure the sweetener. The oil residue on the cup will allow the sticky sweetener to slide out easily. For even baking, unless otherwise instructed in a recipe, bake food on the center oven rack.

» To get the most juice out of fresh lemons, limes, or oranges, roll them against the kitchen countertop before squeezing.
» If you want a chocolate flavor, substitute carob powder for cocoa.
» When using oat flour, make sure it is certified pure oat flour with no possible presence of wheat or gluten. Our recipes generally call for oat flour and brown rice flour, but amaranth, buckwheat, chickpea (garbanzo), millet, potato, quinoa, and teff flours can be substituted in equal amounts.
» When using canned beans, buy organic varieties that are free of salt and make sure the cans are BPA free.
» When it comes to using herbs and spices, it is always best to use fresh when available. If using dried, be sure to check expiration dates. Most dried herbs lose their potency within a few months. Remember this ratio: 1 tablespoon fresh = 1 teaspoon dried.
» Many of the recipes in this book can be made in advance and stored in the refrigerator or freezer.

Now that you are armed with the information you need to prepare brain healthy meals, it's time to get started!

CHAPTER 4

Recipes for Brain Health

Sensational Smoothies
Awesome Appetizers
Splendid Sides
Exceptional Entrees
Spectacular Salads
Super Soups
Delightful Desserts and Snacks

A Few Notes

» For many recipes, we note that you can use a blender or food processor to prepare them. Not everyone has both appliances. For recipes in the Sensational Smoothies section, though, we use a blender.

» Please note the following abbreviations in the recipes: Cup (c.), Tablespoon (T.), teaspoon (tsp.) and Fahrenheit (F).

» Please use extra-virgin olive oil in recipes, as it is extracted using natural methods and standardized for purity and certain sensory qualities like taste and smell.

» You'll see a few recipes that call for vegetables to be steamed as part of the instructions. Steaming is a great way to prepare vegetables. It doesn't require any extra fats, and the gentle heat of steam helps vegetables keep more of their nutrients and flavor. If you don't have a steaming basket, colander, or strainer, you can still steam your vegetables in a big pot. Once your vegetables are in a pot, the key is to add just a bit of water to the bottom (about 1/2 inch) and boil. Once the water boils, turn off the heat and keep the vegetables in the pot, covered, to keep most of the steam in.

SENSATIONAL SMOOTHIES

Smoothies are a healthy, satisfying way to enjoy fruit! And you can whip one up in a matter of minutes! Although the foundation of a basic smoothie is fruit or fruit juice that is often thickened with ice, there are lots of ingredients (and ingredient combinations) that can turn a simple smoothie into a luscious drink with added flavor, richness, and nutritional value. We've listed some of our favorite smoothie ingredients here. Have fun coming up with your own flavorful creations!

Juices to Add

Acai
Apple
Blueberry
Carrot
Cherry
Cranberry
Goji berry
Grape
Grapefruit
Kiwi
Lemon/lime
Mango
Orange
Papaya
Peach
Pear
Pineapple
Pomegranate
Raspberry
Watermelon

Fruits and Veggies to Add (peeled and pitted)

Acai
Apples
Apricots
Avocados
Blueberries
Bell peppers
Blackberries
Cantaloupes
Cranberries
Cucumbers
Dates
Goji berries
Figs
Grapes
Grapefruit
Honeydew
Kale
Kiwis
Lemons/limes
Mangos
Oranges
Papaya
Peaches
Pears
Pineapple
Plums
Pomegranates
Raspberries
Strawberries
Spinach
Watermelon

Thickeners

Soak up the nutrients. We like to soak our raw seeds and nuts because they are easier to digest, and this enhances the nutritional value of the raw seeds and nuts. We suggest soaking them from two to eight hours. Soak them in glass containers and place in refrigerator.

Add Some Thickness

Avocados
Bananas
Ice cubes
Rolled oats, soaked
Raw nuts (e.g., almonds, pecans, cashews, or walnuts soaked)
Raw seeds (e.g., chia, flax, pumpkin or sunflower seeds), soaked
Sorbets

Flavorful Goodies

Acai berries/puree
Carob powder
Cinnamon
Coconut milk
Dates
Ginger
Goji berries
Non-dairy unsweetened milks
Nuts
Pure maple syrup
Raw honey
Seeds
Tea
Turmeric
Unsweetened coconut flakes
Vanilla extract

We prefer unsweetened almond milk in the recipes because it has a naturally sweet flavor and milky texture. However, you can substitute other non-dairy milk of choice, such as hemp, rice, soy, flax, hazelnut, cashew, or oat milk, for almond milk. We have included a simple recipe for almond milk in this chapter.

Supplements

Aloe vera juice (aids digestion)
Bee pollen (nature's mix of 18 amino acids, 14 minerals, enzymes, and all B vitamins)
Brewer's yeast or nutritional yeast (a source of protein and B vitamins, including B12, that reinforces immune system)
Dairy-free protein powder
Emergen-C brand fizz drink powdered packets
Lecithin (helps prevent accumulation of fat and cholesterol)
Nut butters (almond, cashew, peanut, sunflower, and soy)
Oat bran (great source of fiber that helps lower blood cholesterol level)
Organic tofu (nondairy protein source)
Spirulina (a microalgae that is an excellent source of protein, B vitamins, and iron)

Almond Milk
Avocado Mango Shake
Awesome Acai Delight
Banana Bee Smoothie
Berry Creamy Smoothie
Blue and Green Tea Smoothie
Caramel Apple Smoothie
Carob Banana Smoothie
Ginger Pear Smoothie
Green Goddess Smoothie
Honeydew Kiwi Sensation
Mango Lime Smoothie
Maui Sunrise Surprise
Mixed Berry Blast

Monkey Shake
Orange Granola Smoothie
Orange Mango Melody
Raspberry Smoothie
Red Grape Rejuvenator
Strawberry Carob Smoothie
Strawberry Melon Smoothie
Turmeric Turbo Smoothie
Watermelon Shake

Almond Milk

It's easy to make your own almond milk, and it keeps in the refrigerator for two days. We feel the almond milk is sweet enough as is. However, if you wish to make the almond milk sweeter, add 1 T. maple syrup and 1/2 tsp. vanilla extract to the almond milk mixture. The almond milk picks up the flavors of any cereal or granola that you mix it with; that is why we don't feel it is necessary to add additional sweetener.

YIELD: 2 C.

1 c. raw almonds
2 1/4 c. water
Fine-mesh nut bag or cheesecloth
1 T. maple syrup (optional)
1/2 tsp. vanilla extract (optional)

1. Place almonds in a bowl, cover with water (about an inch over the almonds), and soak overnight.
2. Drain almonds in a strainer under cold water.
3. Place in a blender or food processor.
4. Add 2 c. water. Blend until mixture is smooth, about 5 minutes.
5. Place nut bag or cheesecloth over a large bowl.
6. Place mixture into the cheesecloth and squeeze out the liquid into the bowl. Use almond milk immediately or store in the refrigerator.

Avocado Mango Shake

The avocado and coconut yogurt give this drink a creamy consistency that tastes delicious!

YIELD: 2 SERVINGS

1 c. cubed, pitted mango
1 ripe avocado, smashed
12 oz. vanilla-flavored coconut yogurt
2 T. lime juice
12 ice cubes

1. Blend all ingredients together and serve immediately.

CHANGE IT UP: If you are not allergic to nuts, substitute almond milk– or soy milk–flavored yogurt for vanilla-flavored coconut yogurt.

Awesome Acai Delight

Acai (pronounced "ah-SIGH-ee") is a tiny berry that grows on a species of palm tree in Brazil. It is loaded with antioxidants and disease-fighting phytonutrients that are great for the brain! The flavor is often described as a combination of red wine and chocolate. The frozen blueberries give this smoothie a frosty consistency.

YIELD: 1 SERVING

1 c. unsweetened almond milk
1 c. blueberries (frozen preferred)
1 banana
1/2 c. frozen acai berry puree

1. Place almond milk and blueberries in blender.
2. Add banana and frozen acai berries.
3. Blend on high for about 15 seconds or until smooth.

CHANGE IT UP: Add 1/4 c. chopped kale or spinach to get a daily dose of greens!

Banana Bee Smoothie

Freezing the bananas ahead of time makes for a thicker smoothie, but this smoothie can be made with ripe, unfrozen bananas, too.

YIELD: 2–4 SERVINGS

3 bananas, frozen
1 1/2 c. almond milk
1 1/2 c. unsweetened pineapple juice
1/8 tsp. ground nutmeg
1 tsp. vanilla extract
1 T. bee pollen
4 ice cubes

1. Blend all ingredients in a blender to desired consistency. Serve and enjoy!

CHANGE IT UP: Add 1/4 c. unsweetened shredded coconut.

Add 4 Classic Oatmeal Raisin cookies (page 178) to this smoothie. (Add to blender and blend to desired consistency.)

Berry Creamy Smoothie

This smoothie contains chia seeds, which are loaded with healthy omega-3 fats and fiber. Tofu takes on the flavor of the berries and adds protein to this sweet smoothie. Soy is highly processed and most soy is GMO. Therefore we only use "organic" soy products.

YIELD: 2 SERVINGS

1 c. strawberries
1 c. blueberries
1/2 c. cubed organic tofu (firm type)
1 T. chia seeds
1 c. water
4 ice cubes

1. Blend all ingredients in a blender until smooth.

CHANGE IT UP: Substitute 1/2 c. raw cashews for tofu.

Substitute blackberries or raspberries for strawberries.

Blue and Green Tea Smoothie

Decaffeinated green tea combined with the blueberries and spirulina supplies a great dose of daily antioxidants.

YIELD: 2–4 SERVINGS

2 c. decaffeinated green tea, steeped and chilled
2 c. frozen blueberries
2 bananas (frozen preferred)
1/2 c. chopped spinach
2 tsp. spirulina powder
4 ice cubes

1. Blend all ingredients in a blender until smooth.

Caramel Apple Smoothie

Dates and apple give this smoothie a "candy apple" taste, and oats add fiber to make this a rich and delicious smoothie.

YIELD: 2 SERVINGS

2/3 c. gluten-free rolled oats, soaked for an hour and drained of any excess water
1/2 tsp. cinnamon
1/4 tsp. nutmeg
4 pitted dates
2 T. raw cashews
2 Fuji organic apples, chopped
1 c. unsweetend apple juice
1 c. ice cubes

1. Blend all ingredients in a blender until smooth.

CHANGE IT UP: Substitute 2 T. soaked, raw sunflower seeds for cashews.

Carob Banana Smoothie

Carob and almonds are a sweet combination filled with fiber and protein.

YIELD: 2 SERVINGS

1 3/4 c. unsweetened almond milk
1 T. carob powder
2 ripe bananas (fresh or frozen)
2 T. maple syrup or honey
1/4 c. almonds
6 ice cubes

1. Place almond milk in a cup.
2. Stir in carob powder until it dissolves.
3. Place carob almond milk in blender and add bananas, maple syrup or honey, almonds, and ice cubes.
4. Blend until smooth. Serve immediately.

Ginger Pear Smoothie

Figs are high in calcium, fiber, and flavor! You can use unsulfered dried figs if you can't get fresh figs. We recommend soaking dried figs (using the same amout of dried figs for fresh figs) for an hour before blending them into this smoothie.

YIELD: 2 SERVINGS

1 1/2 c. pear juice
2 T. flaxseeds
1 T. chopped fresh ginger
1 banana
2 pears, peeled and cut into 1-inch pieces
1/2 c. chopped figs
4 ice cubes

1. Blend all ingredients in a blender until smooth. Serve immediately.

Green Goddess Goodness

Grapes and apple juice give this super green drink a dab of welcomed sweetness.

YIELD: 4 SERVINGS

1 c. chopped baby spinach leaves
2 c. green seedless grapes
1 medium green apple, chopped
1/2 medium green bell pepper, diced
2 c. apple juice
1 tsp. spirulina powder (optional)

1. Blend all ingredients well in a blender. (Mixture will be slightly pulpy, yet smooth.)

CHANGE IT UP: Substitute romaine lettuce or kale for spinach.

Honeydew Kiwi Sensation

Mint and lime make this green drink super refreshing!

YIELD: 2 SERVINGS

- 2 c. 1-inch cubes peeled and seeded honeydew melon
- 1 1/2 c. 1/2-inch cubes peeled kiwi
- 1 T. lime juice
- 1 T. maple syrup
- 4 fresh mint leaves, chopped
- 2 c. ice cubes

1. Blend all ingredients in a blender until smooth.

CHANGE IT UP: Substitute cantaloupe for honeydew.

Mango Lime Smoothie

We recommend freezing the fruit in this smoothie because it gives the smoothie a creamy, thick texture.

YIELD: 1–2 SERVINGS

- 2 T. lime juice
- 2 frozen bananas
- 1 c. diced frozen mango
- 1 c. almond milk
- 4 ice cubes

1. Blend all ingredients in a blender until smooth.

Maui Sunrise Surprise

Enjoy this tropical drink on a sunny afternoon.

YIELD: 4 SERVINGS

- 1 c. diced fresh pineapple
- 2 frozen bananas
- 1 c. diced, peeled, and seeded papaya
- 2 c. cubed peeled mango
- 1 c. pineapple juice
- 1/2 c. chopped macadamia nuts
- 1 tsp. vanilla extract
- 6 ice cubes

1. Blend all ingredients in a blender until smooth. Serve immediately.

Mixed Berry Blast

Acai puree adds to the berry flavors in this delicious drink. Frozen acai puree is available in the frozen section of most supermarkets.

YIELD: 2 SERVINGS

1/2 c. fresh blackberries
1/2 c. fresh blueberries
1/2 c. fresh raspberries
1/4 c. frozen acai puree
1/2 c. pomegranate or cranberry juice
1 1/2 c. ice cubes

1. Blend all ingredients in a blender until smooth.

Monkey Shake

You'll go bananas over the combination of bananas and peanut butter in this super smoothie!

YIELD: 1 SERVING

1 large frozen banana
4 T. peanut butter
1 c. hemp milk or almond milk
1 T. maple syrup
1 T. flaxseed meal

1. Blend all ingredients in a blender until smooth.

Orange Granola Smoothie

Granola adds a crunchy texture to this sweet drink.

YIELD: 2 SERVINGS

1 c. Cashew Coconut Granola (page 177)
2 bananas (frozen preferred)
1 c. orange juice
6 ice cubes

1. Blend all ingredients in a blender to desired consistency.

Orange Mango Melody

Avocado and almonds give a smooth flavor to this delicious smoothie.

YIELD: 2 SERVINGS

2 c. orange juice
1 c. cut mango cubes (fresh or frozen)
1 Hass avocado, sliced
1 banana
2 T. raw almonds, soaked preferred (soaked at least an hour and with water drained off)
1 T. flaxseeds
6 ice cubes (approximately 1/2 c.)

1. Blend all ingredients in a blender until smooth. Serve immediately.

Raspberry Smoothie

Berry smoothies are great for the brain. Any berry will work for this delicious smoothie.

YIELD: 1 SERVING

1 c. raspberries (frozen or fresh)
1 frozen banana
1 1/2 c. almond milk
1 T. chia seeds
1 tsp. vanilla extract
4 ice cubes

1. Blend all ingredients in a blender until smooth. Serve immediately.

Red Grape Rejuvenator

This smoothie has the benefits of resveratrol, found in grapes, and the sweetness of fabulous fiber found in figs.

YIELD: 2 SERVINGS

5 medium fresh figs
2 c. organic seedless red grapes
1/2 c. chopped romaine lettuce
2 bananas (frozen preferred)
1 1/4 c. water
4 ice cubes

1. Blend all ingredients in a blender until smooth. Serve immediately.

Strawberry Carob Smoothie

Like having chocolate-covered strawberries in a smoothie!

YIELD: 2 SERVINGS

2 c. coconut milk
1 T. coconut oil
1 c. fresh strawberries (or frozen)
1 tsp. vanilla extract
1 banana
1/2 tsp. cinnamon
1 c. ice cubes

1. Blend all ingredients in a blender to desired consistency. Serve immediately.

Strawberry Melon Smoothie

We enjoy serving this smoothie on the 4th of July when watermelon is at its peak of sweetness. Serve this smoothie in chilled glasses!

YIELD: 2 SERVINGS

1 c. quartered strawberries
2 c. cut seedless watermelon
1 1/4 c. white grape juice
1/2 c. ice cubes

1. Blend all ingredients in a blender until smooth. Serve immediately.

Turmeric Turbo Smoothie

Turmeric, cinnamon, coconut, and chia seeds give this smoothie a boost of antioxidants and turmeric helps reduce inflammation in the body.

YIELD: 1 SERVING

1 c. hemp milk or coconut milk
1/2 c. frozen mango chunks
1 banana (frozen preferred)
1 T. coconut oil
1/2 tsp. turmeric
1/2 tsp. cinnamon
1 tsp. chia seeds

1. Place hemp milk in a blender.
2. Add remaining ingredients, and blend until smooth.

Watermelon Shake

Coconut milk gives this simple shake a smooth, sweet flavor.

YIELD: 2 SERVINGS

4 c. chopped seedless watermelon chunks
1/2 c. coconut milk
1/2 c. ice cubes

1. Blend all ingredients in a blender to desired consistency. Serve immediately.

AWESOME APPETIZERS

Avocado and Tomato Salsa
Black Bean, Jalapeno, and Cilantro Dip
Black Bean and Sun-Dried Tomatoes Dip
Carrot Hummus
Celery Boats
Chili-Lime Baked Tortilla Chips
Cucumber Slices With Dill
Cucumber Parsley Relish
Eggplant and Olive Dip
Fava Bean and Mint Hummus
Fresh Basil Pesto
Fresh Red Bell Pepper Hummus
Garlicky Eggplant and Red Bell Pepper Dip
Golden Mashed Potatoes
Great Guacamole
Happening Hummus
Mango Jalapeno Salsa

Avocado and Tomato Salsa

Tomatoes, corn kernels, and fresh avocado give this salsa a delicious, sweet flavor. Try this salsa on top of a bed of greens or on top of Chili-Lime Baked Tortilla Chips. Include the jalapeno seeds if you want more heat.

YIELD: 2 SERVINGS (1 C.)

1 c. cooked corn kernels
1 ripe avocado, peeled and cut into small pieces
2 large tomato, seeded and diced
1 onion, diced
1 jalapeno, finely chopped
2 T. chopped fresh cilantro
1/4 c. lime juice
2 cloves garlic, minced
1 tsp. garlic salt

1. Combine all ingredients in a medium bowl and mix well.
2. Cover and marinate at least 1 hour before serving.

Black Bean, Jalapeno, and Cilantro Dip

Fresh jalapeno chilies add burst of heat to this bean dip. Cilantro complements the chilies to make this a fiesta favorite.

YIELD: 2–4 SERVINGS (APPROXIMATELY 1 1/2 C.)

2 cloves garlic, minced
1/2 c. loosely packed cilantro leaves
2 jalapeno chilies, seeds removed and coarsely chopped
2 T. extra-virgin olive oil
1 15-oz. can black beans, drained and rinsed
1/4 c. lime juice
1 tsp. garlic salt

1. Blend garlic, cilantro leaves, jalapeno chilies, and olive oil in a blender about 20 seconds, or until ingredients looks like a rough puree.
2. Add beans, lime juice, and garlic salt, and blend an additional 20 seconds.
3. Transfer mixture to a bowl and serve.

CHANGE IT UP: Substitute lemon juice for lime juice.
Substitute garbanzo beans for black beans.

Black Bean and Sun-Dried Tomatoes Dip

Black beans are full of fiber, and sun-dried tomatoes make this dip delicious! For time's sake we use canned black beans. However, you can use fresh-cooked black beans. This dip tastes great on top of rice cakes with sliced avocados.

YIELD: 2 SERVINGS (APPROXIMATELY 1 C.)

1 T. extra-virgin olive oil
3 cloves garlic, minced
1 yellow onion, diced
1 14-oz. can sun-dried tomatoes
1 15-oz. can black beans (or 2 c. fresh cooked black beans)
1/4 tsp. sea salt
1 tsp. cumin
1/4 tsp. chili powder

1. Blend all ingredients in a blender until smooth. Serve and enjoy!

Carrot Hummus

This bright orange hummus is high in vitamin A and antioxidants that are great for the brain. It is delicious served with red bell pepper slices and stuffed in the hollow parts of celery.

YIELD: 2 SERVINGS

1 c. chopped carrots
1 15-oz. can organic garbanzo beans, rinsed and drained
1/4 c. sesame seed spread (tahini)
3 T. lemon juice
3 cloves garlic, minced
1/2 tsp. cumin
1/4 tsp. sea salt
1 T. fresh parsley, chopped

1. Steam carrots approximately 5 minutes or until tender.
2. Drain carrots and place in a food processor.
3. Add garbanzo beans, tahini, lemon juice, garlic, cumin, and sea salt, cover, and process until smooth.
4. Mix in parsley.
5. Refrigerate at least 1 hour and then serve.

Celery Boats

Kids especially love this fun finger food. It's a great way for them to enjoy the high minerals and vitamins in celery. Celery adds the perfect amount of moisture when eating almond butter.

YIELD: 4 SERVINGS

8 stalks celery
1 T. cinnamon
3/4 c. almond butter
1/2 c. raisins

1. Cut each celery stalk in half, making a total of 16 pieces.
2. Place celery on a platter with hollow part facing up, and sprinkle evenly with cinnamon.
3. Spoon about 2 T. almond butter into the hollow part of each celery.
4. Top each piece with raisins.

CHANGE IT UP: Substitute sunflower seed butter, cashew butter, or peanut butter for almond butter.

Substitute Happening Hummus for almond butter, garlic salt for cinnamon, and sliced olives for raisins.

Chili-Lime Baked Tortilla Chips

These are fun chips to eat that have some heat to them. These chips can be eaten alone or with salsa, guacamole, or hummus.

YIELD: 2 SERVINGS

10 corn tortillas
2 T. extra-virgin olive oil
2 T. lime juice
1 tsp. chili powder
1 tsp. garlic salt
Dash cayenne pepper

1. Preheat oven to 350 degrees F.
2. Coat tortillas with oil and cut into triangles.
3. Mix lime juice, chili powder, garlic salt, and cayenne in a medium bowl.
4. Brush lime juice mixture onto each chip.
5. Reduce oven temperature to 250 degrees F.
6. Bake 15 minutes, or until crisp.

Cucumber Slices With Dill

This snack is especially refreshing on a hot summer day. Instead of using a fork to pick up these marinated cucumber slices, we recommend toothpicks.

YIELD: 1–2 SERVINGS

1 large cucumber, sliced in rounds
1/4 c. apple cider vinegar
1 tsp. dried dill weed
1/2 tsp. fresh ground black pepper

1. Place cucumbers in a shallow bowl.
2. Pour vinegar over cucumbers.
3. Stir in dill weed and black pepper.
4. Refrigerate at least 1 hour, and serve.

Cucumber Parsley Relish

This is a fun party snack, especially for the 4th of July, when corn and cucumbers are at their peak. This relish can be eaten plain or served on top of rice cakes, with baked chips, or on a bed of lettuce. It will keep in the refrigerator up to a week.

YIELD: 4 SERVINGS

5 large ears corn
1 large yellow onion, finely chopped
2/3 c. diced cucumber
1/4 c. lemon juice
1/4 c. extra-virgin olive oil
2 T. finely chopped parsley
1 tsp. sea salt

1. Remove husks and silk from corn.
2. Fill a large pot with a steamer and bring water to a boil. Place corn in water and cook, covered, 10 minutes.
3. Let corn cool, and slice kernels from the cobs with a sharp knife.
4. In a medium bowl mix corn kernels, onion, and cucumber.
5. Stir in lemon juice, olive oil, parsley, and sea salt. Serve immediately or chill.

CHANGE IT UP: Substitute 1 c. diced pickles for cucumber.

Eggplant and Olive Dip

This dip can be served on top of cucumber slices, in the hollow part of celery stalks, or on top of crackers.

YIELD: 4 SERVINGS

1 large eggplant
8 pitted black olives
1 c. diced tomatoes
1 medium yellow onion, chopped
2 T. finely chopped fresh basil
1/4 c. red wine vinegar or apple cider vinegar
2 T. extra-virgin olive oil
2 cloves garlic, minced
1/2 tsp. garlic powder
1/4 tsp. dried oregano
1/4 tsp. ground black pepper

1. Preheat oven to 350 degrees F.
2. Reduce oven temperature to 250 degrees F.
3. Bake eggplant, on a baking sheet, 1 hour, turning occasionally. Poke eggplant with a fork to make sure it is tender.
4. Remove eggplant from oven and cool on baking sheet.

5. Cut eggplant lengthwise and scoop pulp into a mixing bowl. Discard skin.
6. Place eggplant pulp in a food processor and pulse until smooth.
7. Add black olives and pulse a few seconds.
8. Stir in tomatoes, onion, basil, vinegar, olive oil, garlic, garlic powder, oregano, and black pepper.
9. Cover and chill for 1 hour.

Fava Bean and Mint Hummus

Fava beans contain levodopa (L-DOPA), a precursor of neurochemicals in the brain such as dopamine, epinephrine, and norepinephrine. Dopamine in the brain is associated with smooth functioning of body movements.

YIELD: 2–4 SERVINGS

1 lb. fresh fava beans (shelled weight) (frozen if not in season)
1/4 tsp. sea salt
1/2 c. extra-virgin olive oil
1/4 c. fresh mint, finely chopped
1/4 c. fresh dill
1/4 c. fresh lemon juice

1. Steam fresh beans in lightly salted boiling water until tender (about 5 minutes).
2. Drain beans and plunge into ice-cold water.
3. Slide beans out of their skins, transfer to a blender or food processor, and pulse to form a rough puree. (If using frozen fava beans, put them in cold water to defrost and then slide them from the skins. No cooking is required and color will be a lot more vibrant.)
4. Add olive oil, mint, dill, and lemon juice.
5. Pulse or blend until smooth.

Fresh Basil Pesto

Pesto may seem daunting to make, but it's really quite simple. Traditional pesto uses Parmesan cheese, but we have substituted nutritional yeast. It's delicious and high in B12, which is excellent for the brain. This pesto will keep for five days in the refrigerator. Serve with gluten-free crackers or vegetable sticks.

YIELD: 2 SERVINGS (1/2 C.)

2/3 c. pine nuts
3 cloves garlic, minced
3/4 c. fresh basil leaves
6 green onions (white and green parts)
1/4 c. parsley leaves
2 T. nutritional yeast
2 T. fresh lemon juice
1/4 tsp. sea salt
3 T. extra-virgin olive oil

1. Process pine nuts, garlic, basil, green onions, parsley, nutritional yeast, lemon juice, and sea salt in a food processor until finely minced.
2. With the food processor on, slowly pour in olive oil.
3. Transfer to a small bowl. Serve at room temperature.

CHANGE IT UP: Substitute sunflower seeds or pumpkin seeds for pine nuts.

Fresh Red Bell Pepper Hummus

Red bell pepper is full of flavor and vitamin C. It adds a sweet flavor and beautiful color to this hummus. Serve this hummus with fresh vegetable sticks (carrots, celery, and/or bell pepper), or scoop a Tablespoon. of the mixture in the bed of endive lettuce leaf and sprinkle paprika on top.

YIELD: 2–4 SERVINGS (1 C.)

1 15-oz. can garbanzo beans
2 T. tahini
4 T. extra-virgin olive oil
2 T. lemon juice
2 cloves garlic, minced
1 red bell pepper, seeded and chopped
1/2 tsp. sea salt

1. Drain and rinse garbanzo beans.
2. Blend half of garbanzo beans, tahini, olive oil, lemon juice, garlic, red bell peppers, and sea salt into food processor or blender until smooth.
3. Gradually add remaining garbanzo beans through the cap opening while continuing to blend.

Garlicky Eggplant and Red Bell Pepper Dip

The longer this dip marinates, the tastier is becomes, so we recommend making this dip the night before and refrigerating it. This dip is delicious on top of endive leaves, in the crevice of celery, or on top of baked corn chips.

YIELD: 3 c.

2 medium eggplants (1 1/2 lb.), skin on, halved lengthwise
1 medium yellow onion, skin on, halved
1 T. extra-virgin olive oil
6 large cloves garlic
1/2 c. red bell peppers
1/2 c. lemon juice
1 tsp. cinnamon
1 tsp. sea salt
2 T. minced parsley, for garnish

1. Preheat oven to 350 degrees F.
2. Lightly brush cut sides of eggplants and onion with 1 T. olive oil, and place on a baking sheet, cut side down.
3. Reduce oven temperature to 250 degrees F.
4. Bake eggplant and onion about an hour, or until very tender.
5. Place eggplant in a colander to drain and cool 15 minutes.
6. Scoop out pulp from skins and place in the bowl of a food processor.
7. Add onion, red bell pepper, and garlic.
8. Blend the mixture until smooth.
9. Stir in lemon juice, cinnamon, and sea salt.
10. Place dip in small bowl and garnish with parsley.

Golden Mashed Potatoes

Skip the butter, not the flavor. These mashed potatoes can be served as a side dish or scooped into a leaf of lettuce with sliced olives on top! Yukon gold potatoes are the ideal potatoes to use in this recipe to get a creamy texture.

YIELD: 2–4 SERVINGS

8 large Yukon gold potatoes, peeled and cut into 1-inch pieces
1 c. water
1 c. almond milk
1/4 c. extra-virgin olive oil
1 tsp. garlic salt
1 tsp. sea salt
1/8 tsp. nutmeg
4 green onions, finely sliced
Dash of paprika

1. Steam potatoes with water in a large pot about 20 minutes or until tender.
2. Use a potato ricer or large fork to mash the potatoes.
3. Return mashed potatoes to pot.
4. In a small saucepan, heat the almond milk over medium heat until warm, about 3 minutes.
5. Stir warm almond milk into the mashed potatoes.
6. Stir in olive oil and heat mixture on low heat keeping the mixture warm.
7. Stir in garlic salt, sea salt and nutmeg. Continue to stir ingredients on low heat for another minute.
8. Sprinkle green onions and paprika over potatoes, and serve warm.

Great Guacamole

This guacamole is delicious on tortilla chips, rice cakes, crackers, or a bed of lettuce. We make an effort to not add additional salt to any of the recipes; however, we feel the flavor of this guacamole is truly enhanced by the minimal amount of sea salt.

YIELD: 2–4 SERVINGS

3 ripe avocados, mashed (keep the seed)
1 tomato, diced
1 onion, diced
3 T. lemon juice
1 tsp. sea salt
2 green onions, finely sliced

1. Spoon out avocado into a large bowl.
2. Mash avocado with a fork.
3. Add tomato, onion, lemon juice, sea salt, and green onions to avocado mixture, and stir well. Serve immediately or chill with a tight

plastic wrap on top and put the one avocado seed in the middle to retain color.

CHANGE IT UP: Substitute lime juice for lemon juice for a sweeter flavor. Add 1/4 c. salsa to the guacamole for a fun spicy flavor and texture.

Happening Hummus

Hummus with veggies is a healthy, tasty snack. The natural color and texture are filled with protein, fiber, vitamins, and minerals! Enjoy with pita chips or wrapped in gluten-free tortillas.

YIELD: 4 C.

1/2 c. toasted sesame seed butter (tahini)
1/4 c. warm water
1/4 c. extra-virgin olive oil
1/8 c. lemon juice
2 15-oz. cans garbanzo beans (approximately 2 c.), drained and rinsed
3 cloves minced garlic
1 tsp. ground cumin
1/4 tsp. black pepper
1/2 tsp. sea salt

1. Blend sesame seed butter, water, olive oil, and lemon juice in a blender or food processor 30 seconds.
2. Add garbanzo beans, 1 c. at a time, and blend well.
3. Add garlic, cumin, black pepper, and sea salt.
4. Blend an additional 10 seconds. Cover and refrigerate until ready to serve.

CHANGE IT UP: Add 2 T. fresh salba seeds. Salba is part of the chia seed family. Salba is a natural source of omega-3 fatty acid, and salba has eight times more omega-3s than salmon and four more times than flaxseeds. Omega-3 fatty acids play a crucial role in brain function and heart health. Flaxseeds add a nutty, welcomed flavor and are high in omega-3s also.

Substitute sesame seed oil for olive oil for a nuttier flavor.

Mango Jalapeno Salsa

Mango adds a sweet twist and the jalapenos add a kick to this easy-to-make salsa. This is excellent served cold and can be kept in the refrigerator for five days.

YIELD: 2–4 SERVINGS (2 C.)

6 medium red tomatoes, seeded and diced
1 medium red onion, diced
2 mangos, diced
1/4 c. red wine vinegar or apple cider vinegar
2 jalapenos, seeded and minced
1/2 c. fresh cilantro, chopped
1 tsp. cayenne pepper

1. Combine all ingredients in a large bowl. Serve immediately or refrigerate up to five days.

Mushroom Lentil Poppers With Cashew-Garlic Sauce

These bite-sized snack balls are so much fun to eat by placing a toothpick in them and dipping them into Cashew Garlic Sauce. Making larger patties out of the mixture works great for veggie burger fillings, also. Make the dipping sauce while the poppers are baking.

YIELD: 30 BALLS

Poppers:

2 1/2 c. cooked lentils
1/4 c. sliced mushrooms
1/4 c. salsa
2 T. oat flour
2 cloves garlic, minced
1 T. nutritional yeast
1 tsp. curry powder
1 tsp. sea salt
1 T. extra-virgin olive oil

Dipping Sauce:

1/2 c. raw cashews, soaked at least 4 hours
1/3 c. water
2 garlic cloves, minced
2 T. extra-virgin olive oil
4 T. lemon juice
2 green onions, sliced
1/2 tsp. sea salt

1. Preheat oven to 350 degrees F.
2. Lightly oil a baking sheet and set aside.

3. Pulse lentils, mushrooms, salsa, oat flour, garlic, and nutritional yeast in a blender or food processor about 15 seconds, or until mixture is fairly smooth.
4. Transfer to mixing bowl.
5. Stir in curry powder and salt.
6. Add oil and mix well.
7. Form mixture into 1 1/2 inch balls and arrange on the baking sheet.
8. Reduce oven temperature to 250 degrees F.
9. Bake 30 minutes.
10. Rinse cashews well and place in a food processor.
11. Add water, garlic, olive oil, lemon juice, green onions, and sea salt.
12. Blend until mixture becomes creamy.
13. Dip warm lentil balls into sauce and enjoy!

Red Grape and Tomato Salsa With Fresh Cilantro

This sweet salsa tastes great cupped in butter leaf lettuce or on top of baked tortilla chips and sliced avocado.

YIELD: 2–4 SERVINGS

4 tomatoes, seeded and chopped
1 c. red seedless grapes, halved
1 red onion, diced
2 T. fresh cilantro leaves
2 T. lime juice
2 garlic cloves, minced
1 tsp. sea salt
1 tsp. hot sauce

1. Place tomatoes, grapes, onion, and cilantro leaves in a bowl.
2. Stir in lime juice, garlic, sea salt, and hot sauce.
3. Chill at least 30 minutes. (The longer the mixture marinates the stronger the flavors will be.)

Simple Kale Chips

Kale is high in vitamins K, A, and C. It's a tasty way to get kids to eat greens!

YIELD: 6 SERVINGS

16 oz. kale (1 large bunch), washed, stemmed, and chopped into 1-inch pieces
3 T. extra-virgin olive oil
1 tsp. sea salt

1. Preheat oven to 350 degrees F.
2. Place kale in a large bowl and set aside.
3. Whisk together oil and salt.
4. Pour oil over kale, and toss well.
5. Spread out kale on a baking sheet in a single layer (you may have to do this in batches).
6. Reduce oven temperature to 250 degrees F.
7. Place baking sheet on a rack in the middle of the oven and bake 10 minutes.
8. Toss the chips with a spatula and bake another 5 minutes, until crisp. Serve warm or room temperature.

CHANGE IT UP: Sprinkle chili powder and garlic powder on the chips.

Taquitos With Pinto Beans and Cheddar Shreds

These baked taquitos make a wonderful finger food that everyone can enjoy. You can use fat-free refried beans, or you can cook your own and mash them into a paste-like mixture.

1 16-oz. can refried beans
3/4 c. vegan cheddar cheese (known as shreds)
1 T. lime juice
3 T. diced mild chilies (optional)
24 corn tortillas
4 T. extra-virgin olive oil
Salsa and/or guacamole, for dipping

1. Preheat oven to degrees 350.
2. In a medium bowl mix beans, vegan cheese, chilies, and lime juice.
3. In a large skillet, warm tortillas one at a time, about 2 minutes, or until soft and pliable.
4. Cut tortillas in half.
5. Coat one side of each tortilla with olive oil, and place in a shallow dish.

6. On the dry side of the tortilla, place about 1 T. of the bean mixture and roll it into a cylinder.
7. Repeat process until all tortillas are filled and rolled up.
8. Place rolled-up tortillas lined up next to one another on a greased baking sheet.
9. Place filled tortillas in oven and reduce oven temperature to 250 degrees F.
10. Bake about 15 minutes.
11. Turn over taquitos and bake an additional 10 minutes. Serve warm, with salsa and guacamole.

CHANGE IT UP: Substitute black beans for pinto beans.

White Bean and Fresh Basil Spread

Basil and garlic give this spread the perfect flavor to spread on crackers or veggies. This spread is wonderful scooped into celery or an endive leaf with a dash of paprika sprinkled on top.

YIELD: 2 SERVINGS

1 15-oz. can white beans, rinsed and drained
4 cloves garlic, peeled and chopped
1/2 c. extra-virgin olive oil
6 leaves fresh basil, chopped (approximately 3 T.)
3/4 tsp. sea salt
1/4 tsp. ground black pepper
2 green onions, sliced (for garnish)

1. Blend beans in a food processor 30 seconds or until smooth.
2. Add garlic, oil, basil, sea salt, and ground black pepper, and pulse about 15 seconds. Use a spoon to make sure it blends evenly.
3. Place spread in small bowl and sprinkle sliced green onions on top for garnish. Serve room temperature or chilled.

Zucchini Basil Dip

Zucchini and basil keeps this dip a fresh green color. (Sometimes dips containing avocados alone can turn a brownish color.) This dip tastes great with red bell pepper strips and raw cauliflower.

YIELD: 2–4 SERVINGS

2 large zucchini, grated
4 green onions, thinly sliced
2 Hass avocados
1 T. chopped fresh parsley
2 T. chopped basil
3 cloves garlic, chopped
2 T. extra-virgin olive oil
2 T. lemon juice
3 T. walnuts, chopped
1 tsp. sea salt

1. Place all ingredients in a food processor and blend until smooth.

CHANGE IT UP: Substitute pecans for walnuts.

SPLENDID SIDES

Asparagus With Fresh Basil and Pine Nuts
Best Baked Vegan Potato Latkes
Cauliflower Bakes
Dijon Brussels Sprouts
Green Bean Casserole
Maple Pecan Butternut Squash With Currants
Mushrooms, Potatoes, and Walnuts With Basil
Quinoa With Tomatoes and Walnuts
Red Potato Cheese Bakes
Sage Cannellini Beans With Mushrooms and Hazelnuts
Sesame Orange-Laced Soba Noodles
Sweetly Glazed Carrots
Tomato-Stuffed Portobellos With Pine Nuts
Yam Baked Fries

Asparagus With Fresh Basil and Pine Nuts

We like to eat seasonally as the produce is at its peak in flavor and nutrition. We look forward to springtime vegetables, which include asparagus. This chilled dish makes an ideal side dish.

YIELD: 2 SERVINGS

1 lb. asparagus, ends cut off and sliced on the diagonal into 1/2-inch slices
2 T. sesame oil
2 T. apple cider vinegar
1 T. pure maple syrup
1/4 c. fresh chopped basil
1/2 tsp. mixed dried Italian herbs
2 T. pine nuts, for garnish

1. Place asparagus into boiling water and cook 2 minutes.
2. Drain asparagus and immediately pat dry.
3. Place asparagus in medium bowl.
4. In a small bowl mix sesame oil, vinegar, maple syrup, basil, and Italian herbs.
5. Pour oil and vinegar mixture over asparagus, and mix well.
6. Refrigerate at least 1 hour. Garnish with pine nuts.

CHANGE IT UP: Substitute sesame seeds or flaxseeds for pine nuts.

Best Baked Vegan Potato Latkes

Traditionally potato latkes, also known as potato pancakes, use matzo meal (made from wheat flour) and eggs. However, these are just as tasty and healthier for you! Potato latkes can be served with unsweetened apple sauce, vegan sour cream, or homemade tomato sauce.

YIELD: 12 PANCAKES

2 Russet potatoes, peeled and grated
1 medium yellow onion, grated
4 T. oat flour or brown rice flour
1 tsp. sea salt
1/8 tsp. black pepper
2 T. extra-virgin olive oil

1. Preheat oven to 350 degrees F.

2. Place grated potatoes on top of a towel or paper towel and squeeze as much water out as possible to get the potatoes as dry as possible.
3. In a large bowl, mix potatoes, onions, oat flour, sea salt, and pepper well.
4. Spoon about 3 T. of the mixture into your hands, make a round patty (about 3x3 inches), place on greased cookie sheet, and press down a little on patty.
5. Repeat process with remaining mixture.
6. Reduce oven temperature to 250 degrees F.
7. Bake 20 minutes per side, using a spatula to turn patties. Serve hot.

Cauliflower Bakes

This is a fun and different way to eat cauliflower. Cauliflower is a member of the cruciferous vegetable family, and it is known for its cancer-preventing nutrients, as well as being high in vitamin C.

YIELD: 4 SERVINGS

1 head cauliflower
2 T. extra-virgin olive oil
2 T. lemon juice
2 tsp. Dijon mustard
1 tsp. sea salt
4 cloves garlic, minced
2 T. nutritional yeast

1. Preheat oven to 350 degrees F.
2. Separate cauliflower into bite-sized florets, and place in a medium bowl.
3. In another medium bowl, whisk olive oil, lemon juice, Dijon mustard, sea salt, minced garlic, and nutritional yeast.
4. Toss cauliflower with oil and lemon dressing.
5. Spread cauliflower on baking sheet.
6. Reduce heat to 250 degrees F.
7. Bake cauliflower 30 minutes. Serve warm.

Dijon Brussels Sprouts

Dijon mustard and maple syrup add a perfect balance of salt and sweetness to the Brussels sprouts.

YIELD: 4 SERVINGS

2 T. extra-virgin olive oil
2 cloves garlic, minced
2 T. Dijon mustard
3 T. maple syrup
1/2 tsp. sea salt
1/4 tsp. ground black pepper
4 c. Brussels sprouts, ends trimmed and sliced in half length-wise
2/3 c. sliced almonds

1. Preheat oven to 350 degrees F.
2. In small bowl, stir oil, garlic, Dijon mustard, maple syrup, sea salt, and pepper well.
3. In a medium bowl place Brussels sprouts, and pour Dijon marinade on top.
4. Stir Brussels sprouts and marinade.
5. Place Brussels sprouts in a single layer on a greased baking sheet.
6. Reduce oven temperature to 250 degrees F.
7. Bake Brussels sprouts 30–35 minutes. Serve immediately.

Green Bean Casserole

This casserole is a big hit at our vegetarian Thanksgivings. For convenience, you can use canned French beans, but if you can get them fresh, it's even better!

YIELD: 4 SERVINGS

1/4 c. extra-virgin olive oil
1/4 c. brown rice flour
1 1/2 c. Classic Vegetable Stock (page 155)
1 tsp. sea salt
1/4 tsp. black pepper
1 tsp. garlic powder
2 cloves garlic, minced
1/4 c. nutritional yeast
2 14.5-oz. cans French-style green beans, drained (or 2 c. fresh green beans)
1/2 c. almonds, slivered

1. Preheat oven to 350 degrees F.
2. In a medium saucepan, warm olive oil over low heat.
3. Add flour and whisk continuously for about 2 minutes.
4. Add vegetable stock, sea salt, black pepper, garlic powder, and minced garlic, whisking continuously 2 minutes, until sauce is thick and bubbly.
5. Add nutritional yeast, and stir until smooth.
6. Pour sauce into a small casserole dish, add green beans, and stir to coat.
7. Reduce oven temperature to 250 degrees F.
8. Bake 15 minutes.
9. Top with slivered almonds and serve warm.

CHANGE IT UP: Substitute hazelnuts or pine nuts for almonds.

Maple Pecan Butternut Squash With Currants

Pure maples syrup, pecans, and currants bring a sensational, sweet flavor to butternut squash.

YIELD: 4 SERVINGS

1/4 c. pure maple syrup
2 T. extra-virgin olive oil
1/2 tsp. sea salt
1 tsp. cinnamon
1 tsp. thyme, dried
1 medium butternut squash, peeled and cubed
1/3 c. currants
2/3 c. coarsely chopped pecans

1. Preheat oven to 350 degrees F.
2. Lightly oil a baking sheet.
3. In a medium bowl mix maple syrup, olive oil, sea salt, cinnamon, and thyme.
4. Add butternut squash, and toss well.
5. Spread squash on baking sheet in a single layer.
6. Reduce oven temperature to 250 degrees F.
7. Bake 50 minutes or until squash is tender.
8. Remove squash and place on a platter.
9. Sprinkle currants and pecans on top, and serve.

Mushrooms, Potatoes, and Walnuts With Basil

Garlic, extra-virgin olive oil, and basil give this dish an Italian flair. Walnuts add a delightful crunch and meaty flavor to the potatoes. It's delicious served warm or chilled.

YIELD: 4 SERVINGS

2 T. plus 3 T. extra-virgin olive oil
3 large russet potatoes, thinly sliced
1/2 tsp. sea salt
4 cloves garlic, minced
1/2 tsp. dried basil
12 medium white or brown mushrooms, thinly sliced
1/2 c. finely chopped walnuts

1. Preheat oven to 350 degrees F.
2. Pour 2 T. olive oil in the bottom of a 9-inch square baking dish. Tilt the dish to distribute the oil evenly.
3. Lay thinly sliced potatoes on the bottom of the baking dish.
4. Sprinkle potatoes with half of sea salt, garlic, and basil.
5. Layer mushrooms and walnuts on top of potatoes and seasonings.
6. Drizzle remaining 3 T. olive oil over mushrooms and walnuts.
7. Sprinkle remaining garlic salt, garlic, and basil over mushrooms.
8. Reduce oven temperature to 250 degrees F.
9. Bake 40 minutes. Serve warm.

Quinoa With Tomatoes and Walnuts

The fluffy, creamy texture of quinoa complimented by the sweet flavor of the tomatoes and nutty flavor of the walnuts makes this a tasty side dish!

YIELD: 4-6 SERVINGS

2 c. quinoa
4 c. water
2/3 c. sliced olives
1 c. finely chopped green onions
2 celery stalks, diced
1/3 c. diced red bell pepper
12 sugar plum tomatoes
2 T. finely chopped parsley
4 T. extra-virgin olive oil
4 T. apple cider vinegar
2 cloves garlic, minced
1/2 tsp. sea salt
2/3 c. walnuts, chopped

1. Rinse quinoa with cold water and strain it.
2. In a pot bring 4 c. water to boil and add quinoa. Reduce to a simmer.
3. Cook about 20 minutes, or until water is absorbed.
4. Place quinoa in a large bowl.
5. Stir in olives, green onions, celery, bell pepper, tomatoes, and parsley.
6. In a small bowl whisk olive oil, vinegar, garlic, and sea salt.
7. Stir olive oil and vinegar mixture into quinoa mixture.
8. Sprinkle walnuts on top and serve.

Red Potato Cheese Bakes

These patties taste great dipped in organic ketchup or wrapped in lettuce.

YIELD: 4 SERVINGS

2 lb. red potatoes
2 medium yellow onions, finely chopped
3 T. chopped parsley
4 T. brown rice flour
2 cloves garlic, minced
1 tsp. sea salt
2 T. water
1/2 c. vegan cheddar cheese

1. Preheat oven to 350 degrees F.
2. Steam potatoes in their skin 30 minutes (until very soft).
3. Cube potatoes and put in a blender.
4. Add onions, parsley, flour, garlic, sea salt, and water.
5. Blend until smooth.
6. Place mixture into a medium bowl and stir in vegan cheddar cheese.
7. Scoop a large T. of mixture and form a patty.
8. Place patty on a lightly oiled baking sheet.
9. Repeat with remaining mixture.
10. Reduce oven temperature to 250 degrees F.
11. Bake 25 minutes. Serve warm.

Sage Cannellini Beans With Mushrooms and Hazelnuts

Fresh sage adds a delicate flavor to the creamy, rich taste of the white beans. This tastes great alone or with vegan mozzarella cheese melted on top. For the beans this recipe calls for, you can use a 15-ounce can of white beans, or you can soak beans overnight and then cook them two hours. For the tomato sauce, use your favorite marinara or use Quick and Easy Tomato.

Yield: 2–4 servings

1 cup sliced white mushrooms
2 c. cannellini beans, picked and rinsed
2 T. chopped fresh sage
2 stalks celery, diced
1 small yellow onion, diced
3 cloves garlic, minced
1 c. tomato sauce
1/4 tsp. ground black pepper
1/2 c. hazelnuts

1. Cook mushrooms, beans, sage, celery, onion, garlic, tomato sauce, and black pepper in medium pot over low heat about 15 minutes, stirring occasionally.
2. Stir in hazelnuts, and serve warm.

Sesame Orange-Laced Soba Noodles

Orange juice combined with balsamic vinegar gives this a tangy, welcoming flavor.

Yield: 2 servings

1/2 lb. buckwheat noodles (soba noodles)
1/4 c. extra-virgin olive oil
1/4 c. balsamic vinegar
1/3 c. orange juice
2 oranges peeled, sectioned, and chopped
2 cloves garlic, minced
1 medium red onion, chopped
1/4 tsp. black pepper
1/4 tsp. cinnamon
1/4 c. sesame seeds
2 tsp. anise seed crushed (optional)

1. Cook noodles according to package directions.
2. Drain noodles under cold water and place in large bowl.

3. Stir in olive oil, vinegar, orange juice, oranges, garlic, onion, black pepper, cinnamon, sesame seeds, and anise seed into noodles until well coated. Serve.

Sweetly Glazed Carrots

Adding honey to steamed carrots enhances their natural sweet flavor. This is a simple and impressive snack.

Yield: 2 servings

2 c. coarsely chopped carrots
2 T. honey
1 tsp. sea salt
1 T. finely chopped fresh dill (or 1/2 tsp. dried)

1. Steam carrots about 10 minutes in a medium pot.
2. Place steamed carrots in a bowl.
3. Add honey, sea salt, and dill.
4. Stir and serve.

Change it up: Substitute pure maple syrup for honey (to make this vegan).

Tomato-Stuffed Portobellos With Pine Nuts

Tomato filling makes a sweet and delicious stuffing for Portobello mushrooms.

Yield: 6 servings

3/4 c. chopped tomatoes
4 T. extra-virgin olive oil, divided
1 tsp. finely chopped fresh oregano
1/4 tsp. ground black pepper
4 cloves garlic, minced
3 T. fresh lemon juice
1 T. balsamic vinegar
6 Portobello mushrooms (5–6 inches in diameter), stems and gills removed
1 T. chopped fresh basil
1/2 c. toasted pine nuts

1. Preheat oven to 350 degrees F.
2. In a small bowl, combine tomatoes, 1 tsp. olive oil, oregano, pepper, and garlic.

3. In another small bowl, whisk remaining olive oil, lemon juice, and vinegar.
4. Using a pastry brush, brush oil-lemon juice mixture on both sides of mushroom caps.
5. Place mushrooms, stem-down, on an oiled baking sheet.
6. Reduce oven temperature to 250 degrees F.
7. Bake 12 minutes.
8. Spoon tomato mixture into each mushroom cap and bake 5 more minutes.
9. Sprinkle with basil and pine nuts, and serve.

Yam Baked Fries

Yams and sweet potatoes are colorful fries that kids and adults love to snack on. Who knew fries could be healthy?

YIELD: 4 SERVINGS

1 lb. yams, peeled and cut into 1/2-inch-thick strips
1 lb. sweet potatoes, peeled and cut into 1/2-inch-thick strips
1 T. honey
1 tsp. cinnamon
3 T. extra-virgin olive oil

1. Preheat oven to 350 degrees F.
2. Toss yams and sweet potatoes in a bowl with honey, cinnamon, and olive oil.
3. Place on a baking sheet in a single layer.
4. Reduce oven temperature to 250 degrees F.
5. Bake 20 minutes.
6. Let cool, and serve.

CHANGE IT UP: Substitute russet or red potatoes for yams and sweet potatoes.

Substitute garlic salt (sprinkled on top) for cinnamon and honey.

EXCEPTIONAL ENTREES

Basil Macaroni Casserole
Bean and Bell Pepper Burgers
Bueno Bean Tacos
Chickpea Coconut Curry
Fresh Lemon and Basil Spaghetti
Ginger Mint Spirals With Pine Nuts
Italian Baked Eggplant
Marvelous Mac and Cheese With Cauliflower
Nona's Pizza
Perfect Pizza Crust
Quick and Easy Pizza Sauce
Polenta Avocado Casserole
Polenta With Acorn Squash and Walnuts
Power Pinto Patties
Quick-Version Macaroni and Cheese
Quinoa Pasta With Mushrooms and Asparagus
Quinoa Walnut Burgers
Satisfying Vegetable Stew
Springtime Pasta Primavera
Sweet Potato Chili
Tomato Spaghetti Squash With Mushrooms
Veggie Lo Mein
Veggie Sushi Supreme
Walnut Tacos With Romaine Wrap

Basil Macaroni Casserole

This baked dish is similar to a lasagna. It can be served warm or cold.

YIELD: 4 SERVINGS

4 c. water
2 c. gluten-free elbow pasta (macaroni style)
2 T. extra-virgin olive oil
1 c. sliced mushrooms
1/4 c. diced celery
1 yellow onion, chopped
3 cloves garlic, minced
1 c. tomato sauce
3 T. chopped fresh basil (or 1 T. dried)
2 c. (8-oz. packet) vegan mozzarella cheese (shreds)

1. Preheat oven to 350 degrees F.
2. In a large pot, boil water.
3. Add pasta to boiling water.
4. Reduce heat to a simmer, and cook pasta 12–15 minutes. (Check cooking instructions on pasta box because over-cooking gluten-free pasta can make it mushy.)
5. Drain pasta under cold water and place in a large bowl.
6. Mix olive oil, mushrooms, celery, onion, and garlic into pasta.
7. Add tomato sauce, basil, and 1 3/4 c. vegan mozzarella cheese.
8. Place the mixture into a 6x8-inch casserole dish.
9. Sprinkle remaining vegan mozzarella cheese on top.
10. Reduce oven temperature to 250 degrees F.
11. Bake 35 minutes.

CHANGE IT UP: Add 1/2 c. peas and chopped broccoli.
Substitute soup of choice for tomato sauce.

Bean and Bell Pepper Burgers

The combination of cilantro and cumin gives these tasty burgers a warm, earthy taste. This mixture can be pre-made and stored in the refrigerator for 24 hours.

YIELD: 4 BURGERS

1 T. extra-virgin olive oil
1/4 c. diced red bell pepper
6 green onions (scallions), sliced
1 stalk celery, chopped
2 cloves garlic, peeled and cut in quarters
1 15-oz. can black beans
1 T. chopped fresh cilantro
1/4 c. oat flour
1 T. cumin
1/2 tsp. sea salt

1. Preheat oven to 350 degrees F.
2. In a large skillet stir olive oil, bell pepper, green onions, celery, and garlic over low heat 2 minutes.
3. Rinse black beans with water.
4. Process beans in a food processor or blender about 45 seconds.
5. Add veggie mixture and cilantro, and blend another 15 seconds. (At any time you can stop the blender and stir with a spoon evenly distribute ingredients. The veggies should still be apparent and diced-looking in the mixture.)
6. Transfer bean mixture to a large bowl.
7. Stir in oat flour, cumin, and sea salt.
8. Form 3x3-inch patties and place on an oiled cookie sheet.
9. Reduce oven temperature to 250 degrees F.
10. Cook each side of burger about 10 minutes.

Bueno Bean Tacos

These tasty tacos are filled with sweet corn and fiber-rich black beans.

YIELD: 4 TACOS

1 c. cooked black beans
1 c. cooked corn kernels (preferably fresh)
1/2 c. salsa
2 cloves garlic, minced
1 small red onion, diced
1/4 c. cilantro, chopped
1 tsp. cumin
1/4 tsp. black pepper
1/8 tsp. cayenne pepper
4 corn tortillas
1/2 c. romaine lettuce, chopped
1/2 c. sliced black olives

1. Preheat oven to 350 degrees F.

2. In a medium saucepan stir beans, corn, salsa, garlic, onions, cilantro, cumin, black pepper, and cayenne pepper over low heat about 5 minutes.
3. Place tortillas on a baking sheet.
4. Reduce heat to 250 degrees F.
5. Bake about 10 minutes, or until tortillas are soft enough to fold.
6. Fill each tortilla with 2 scoops of bean mixture.
7. Add desired amount of lettuce and black olives to each tortilla. Serve warm.

Chickpea Coconut Curry

Chickpeas are also known as garbanzo beans. This dish tastes great with fresh or steamed cauliflower.

YIELD: 8–10 SERVINGS

1 15-oz. can coconut milk
4 c. water
2 c. basmati rice
4 cloves garlic, minced
1 c. finely chopped carrots
1 medium red potato, chopped into small cubes
1 15-oz. can chickpeas, drained and rinsed
1 c. fresh corn (or frozen)
1 c. fresh sweet peas (or frozen)
3 T. curry seasoning
1 T. gluten-free soy sauce
1/4 c. lime juice
3 T. finely chopped fresh cilantro

1. In a large pot, bring coconut milk, water, basmati rice, garlic, chopped carrots, potato cubes, chickpeas, corn, and peas to a boil, then reduce heat to a simmer.
2. Cook about 20 minutes.
3. Stir in curry, soy sauce, lime juice, and cilantro.
4. Cook an additional 5 minute, and serve warm.

Fresh Lemon and Basil Spaghetti

Extra-virgin olive oil, lemon, and basil are the perfect combination of enhancing flavors for this spaghetti.

YIELD: 4 SERVINGS

1 lb. rice spaghetti (or any gluten-free spaghetti)
3/4 c. extra-virgin olive oil, divided
1 yellow onion, diced
6 garlic cloves, peeled and finely chopped
1 c. sliced mushrooms
1/4 c. chopped fresh basil
2 T. grated lemon zest (about 4 lemons)
1 tsp. sea salt
2 T. fresh lemon juice
1/2 c. vegan mozzarella shreds

1. Bring a large pot of water to a boil over high heat.
2. Add spaghetti and cook, stirring often to ensure it doesn't stick together, about 12 minutes, or until tender but still firm to the bite.
3. Drain spaghetti.
4. Heat a large, heavy skillet over low heat.
5. Cook 1/2 c. oil, onion, and garlic and about 30 seconds, or just until fragrant.
6. Stir in mushrooms and basil.
7. Add lemon zest and sea salt.
8. Add spaghetti and remaining 1/4 c. oil, and toss to coat.
9. Stir in lemon juice, followed by half of the vegan cheese.
10. Divide pasta among four pasta bowls.
11. Top with the remaining cheese, and serve.

Ginger Mint Spirals With Pine Nuts

Mint and ginger add a spicy, refreshing flavor to this pasta. Pine nuts are a perfect sweet and delicate topping.

YIELD: 4–6 SERVINGS

16 oz. brown rice spiral pasta or gluten-free pasta of your choice
1/4 c. extra-virgin olive oil
1/4 c. chopped green onions
2 cloves garlic, halved
1/4 c. chopped mint leaves
1 T. diced fresh ginger (or 1 tsp. dried)
1/2 c. lemon juice
1 tsp. sea salt
1/2 c. pine nuts

1. Cook pasta according to package directions.
2. Drain pasta and return to pot.

3. In a blender or food processor, blend oil, green onions, garlic, mint leaves, ginger, and lemon juice until mixture becomes a smooth sauce.
4. Pour sauce over pasta in pot and warm 5 minutes.
5. Stir in salt and continue to stir mixture while cooking.
6. Top with pine nuts, and serve warm.

CHANGE IT UP: Substitute soba noodles for rice pasta.

Italian Baked Eggplant

Sprinkling eggplant with salt before cooking draws out the vegetable's moisture and enhances the flavor. This is especially so with larger eggplants because they have more seeds.

YIELDS: 4 SERVINGS

2 medium eggplants
1/2 tsp. sea salt
2 slices rice bread
2 T. almond milk
4 cloves garlic, minced
1 T. minced capers
1 bunch parsley (about 1/2 c.)
1/2 c. black olives (pitted)
2 T. extra-virgin olive oil
2 medium tomatoes, diced
1 tsp. oregano
1/2 tsp. ground black pepper

1. Preheat oven to 350 degrees F.
2. Halve eggplants, score diagonally, salt them, and let sit for 1 hour.
3. Soak rice bread in almond milk.
4. Wash and pat dry eggplant haves and place in an oven-proof dish.
5. In a food processor, blend garlic, capers, parsley, olives, and bread until it becomes a fairly smooth paste.
6. Add olive oil.
7. Spread paste over eggplant halves.
8. Layer eggplants with diced tomatoes.
9. Sprinkle oregano and black pepper on the top of tomatoes.
10. Reduce oven temperature to 250 degrees F.
11. Bake for 1 hour, and serve warm.

Marvelous Mac and Cheese With Cauliflower

The choline found in cauliflower helps improve learning and cognitive function. This cruciferous, powerhouse veggie brings a delightful flavor to this delicious vegan mac and cheese dish. (If you are in a hurry, see the Quick-Version Mac and Cheese on page 115)

YIELD: 4 SERVINGS

4 c. gluten-free elbow macaroni
1 1/2 c. cauliflower, chopped
1/3 c. extra-virgin olive oil
1/3 c. water
1 T. lemon juice
1/2 c. nutritional yeast
2 cloves garlic, minced
1 tsp. sea salt
1/4 tsp. black pepper
Dash of paprika

1. Cook pasta according to package directions.
2. Drain pasta under cold water and set aside.
3. Steam cauliflower about 7 minutes, or until softened.
4. Drain cauliflower.
5. Blend drained cauliflower well in a food processor.
6. Add oil, water, lemon juice, nutritional yeast, garlic, sea salt and pepper, and blend well.
7. Place sauce in a large pot.
8. Add cooked pasta and warm over low-medium heat 5 minutes, stirring frequently.
9. Garnish with a dash of paprika, and serve warm.

CHANGE IT UP: Blend 1/2 c. steamed broccoli into sauce.
Stir in 1/2 c. vegan parmesan cheese before serving.

Nona's Pizza

This gluten-free pizza crust is perfect; you won't miss the wheat! We love to use the Quick and Easy Pizza Sauce, as it is a family recipe created by our grandmother Giovanna, aka Nona. You can use the Quick and Easy Pizza Sauce, a simple basil pesto, or even a simple wipe of olive oil for a base. We like to use fresh vegetables, legumes, herbs, and spices on our pizza. Here are a few terrific topping suggestions:

Artichoke hearts
Asparagus tips
Avocados
Basil
Bell peppers (all colors)
Black beans
Broccoli florets
Capers
Cherry tomatoes
Chickpeas
Eggplant
Fennel
Garlic
Kale
Mushrooms
Olives
Onions
Oregano
Rosemary
Scallions
Spinach
Sun-dried tomatoes
Tomatoes
Zucchini

Perfect Pizza Crust

When you dissolve yeast in the water-honey mixture, it should bubble up and foam within a minute or so. If it doesn't, the yeast is not good. Discard it and start over with fresh yeast. Coating the dough with oil will keep it from drying out. (You can use the same bowl you used to mix the ingredients, and you don't have to clean it first.)

YIELD: 4 THIN CRUSTS (10-INCH ROUNDS)

2 1/4 tsp. active dry yeast (1/4-oz. packet)
1 1/2 c. warm (not hot) water, divided
1 tsp. honey
2 T. extra-virgin olive oil
1 1/2 tsp. dried Italian seasoning blend
1 tsp. sea salt
2 c. brown rice flour
1 1/2 c. tapioca flour

1. Dissolve yeast in a cup or small bowl with 1/2 c. of the warm water and the honey.
2. Transfer the dissolved yeast to a large mixing bowl along with the remaining warm water, oil, Italian seasoning blend, and salt.
3. Stir well with a wooden spoon.
4. Add 1 c. of the brown rice flour and stir well.
5. Continue to stir while adding the remaining brown rice flour and the tapioca flour. When the dough becomes too stiff to stir and starts pulling away from the sides of the bowl, it's time to knead.
6. Turn dough (it will be sticky) onto a clean surface that has been sprinkled with rice flour.

7. Knead dough 4 or 5 minutes, while continuing to sprinkle with flour until dough is smooth and no longer sticky.
8. Place dough in a large, well-oiled bowl, then turn it over so the top is coated with oil.
9. Cover the bowl with a clean, damp dishtowel or plastic wrap.
10. Place in a warm spot about 30 minutes, or until the dough doubles in bulk.
11. Preheat the oven to 350 degrees F.
12. Lightly oil a baking sheet and set aside.
13. Punch down the risen dough, fold it over a few times, then let rest a minute.
14. Divide dough into four equal pieces and shape into balls.
15. Place each ball between sheets of waxed paper and roll out to 10-inch circles about 1/8 inch thick. Pinch the edges with your fingers to create a slightly raised border.
16. Reduce oven temperature to 250 degrees F.
17. Place the rounds on prepared baking sheet and bake 10–15 minutes.
18. Remove from oven, add desired toppings, then return to oven an additional 15–20 minutes, or until the bottom of the crust is browned.

CHANGE IT UP: For added crunch, sprinkle the oiled baking sheet with a handful of cornmeal before adding the dough.

For dough that is a bit flaky and doesn't rise as much, substitute oat flour for brown rice/tapioca flour combo.

Spread sauce and toppings on gluten-free tortillas for a Mexican-themed pizza.

Spread sauce and toppings on top of scooped-out large Portobello mushrooms.

Quick and Easy Pizza Sauce

Our Nona used this simple tomato sauce for pizza and for all pasta dishes, too. The longer it simmers, the thicker it will get and the less acidic it will taste. Use immediately, refrigerate in an airtight container up to a week, or freeze up to six months.

Yield: about 4 c.

3 T. extra-virgin olive oil
1 medium yellow onion, diced
1 clove garlic, minced
1 29-oz. can tomato purée
1 28-oz. can crushed tomatoes
1 T. honey (or maple syrup)
1 T. dried Italian herb seasoning
1 T. dried basil
1/2 tsp. sea salt

1. Heat oil in a large pot over low heat.
2. Add onion and garlic, and sauté less than 5 minutes.
3. Add all remaining ingredients and stir well.
4. Increase heat to medium-high and bring sauce to a boil.
5. Reduce heat to low and simmer uncovered, stirring often, at least 30 minutes, or until sauce reaches the desired consistency.

Polenta Avocado Casserole

This Mexican casserole dish is always a hit at family gatherings! Polenta can be found in the refrigerated section of the store or on the shelves. Either will work.

Yield: 10–12 servings

2 T. extra-virgin olive oil
1 medium onion, chopped (approx. 1/2 c.)
1 medium red bell pepper, chopped
4 cloves garlic, minced
1 15-oz. can black beans, rinsed and drained
1 1/2 c. diced tomatoes
1 c. salsa
3 T. chili powder
1 T. ground cumin
1/4 tsp. cayenne pepper
2 16-oz. tubes cooked polenta
2 c. dairy-free cheddar cheese (We use Daiya Cheddar Shreds.)
1/4 c. chopped fresh cilantro
2 ripe Hass avocados, sliced

1. Preheat oven to 350 degrees F.
2. Put oil in a medium skillet.
3. Cook onion, bell pepper, and garlic in oil over low heat less than 5 minutes.
4. Add beans, tomatoes, salsa, chili powder, cumin, and cayenne and cook about 10 minutes, stirring consistently.
5. Grease a 3-quart rectangular baking dish.

6. Cut one cube of polenta into 1/2-inch cubes and press evenly into prepared baking dish.
7. Halve the second tube of polenta lengthwise and cut into 1/2-inch slices. Set aside.
8. Sprinkle 1 c. cheese over polenta in baking dish.
9. Top with bean mixture.
10. Arrange sliced polenta over bean mixture.
11. Sprinkle with remaining cheese.
12. Reduce oven temperature to 250 degrees F.
13. Bake 45 minutes and sprinkle with cilantro.
14. Let stand about 10 minutes before serving.
15. Place avocado slices over the whole casserole before serving.

Polenta With Acorn Squash and Walnuts

Acorn squash is high in folic acid, which helps maintain brain health.

YIELD: 2 SERVINGS

2 medium acorn squash, halved and seeds removed
2 T. coconut oil, divided
1 yellow onion, chopped
2 cloves garlic, minced
1/4 c. sliced celery
3 c. almond milk
1 c. polenta
1 c. chopped walnuts
1 tsp. black pepper
1 tsp. sage
1/2 tsp. thyme
1/2 tsp. rosemary
1/4 tsp. sea salt

1. Preheat oven to 350 degrees F.
2. Lightly oil squash with 1 T. coconut oil and place cut side down, in an oiled baking pan.
3. Reduce oven temperature to 250 degrees F.
4. Bake squash 45 minutes or until soft.
5. While squash is baking, prepare the polenta stuffing by placing remaining 1 T. coconut oil in a medium saucepan.
6. Add onions, garlic, and celery, and cook over low heat about 3 minutes.
7. Add almond milk and polenta.
8. Increase heat to medium-low while stirring ingredients.
9. Cook about 15 minutes as the mixture begins to thicken.

10. Remove from stovetop and stir in walnuts, black pepper, sage, thyme, rosemary, and sea salt.
11. Remove squash from the oven, and turn over so that the cut side faces up.
12. Fill each half with equal amounts of polenta mixture.
13. Return to oven and bake another 15 minutes. Serve warm.

CHANGE IT UP: Substitute an equal amount of coconut milk for almond milk.

Substitute sunflower or pumpkin seeds for walnuts.

Sprinkle non-dairy parmesan or mozzarella cheese on top of each squash before serving.

Power Pinto Patties

These delicious veggie burgers are wonderful wrapped up in a large lettuce leaf with tomato, red onion, and pickles, or crumbled on top of a salad.

YIELD: 10 PATTIES

2 c. cooked pinto beans, rinsed and drained (canned or fresh cooked)
1/4 c. brown rice flour
1 yellow onion, diced
2 stalks celery, diced
1/2 c. chopped mushrooms
1/2 c. sunflower seeds
2 cloves garlic, minced
1 T. cumin
1/4 tsp. ginger (optional)
1 tsp. sea salt

1. Preheat oven to 350 degrees F.
2. Blend pinto beans in a food processor about 40 seconds, or until smooth.
3. Add rice flour, onion, celery, mushrooms, sunflower seeds, garlic, cumin, ginger, and salt.
4. Pulse until chunky.
5. Scoop small handfuls of the mixture and form into 2- to 3-inch patties about 1/2-inch thick.
6. Place patties on a slightly greased baking sheet.
7. Reduce oven temperature to 250 degrees F.
8. Bake 15 minutes on each side, and serve warm or room temperature.

Quick-Version Macaroni and Cheese

This mac and cheese can also be stored in refrigerator for up to five days.

YIELD: 2–4 SERVINGS

- 8 oz. (approx. 3 c.) rice elbow pasta
- 2 T. vegan margarine (Earth Balance)
- 1 T. extra-virgin olive oil
- 1 T. nutritional yeast
- 1/8 tsp. fresh ground black pepper
- 1 c. almond milk
- 2 c. vegan cheddar cheese (shreds)
- Paprika, for garnish

1. Cook pasta according to package directions.
2. Drain pasta under cold water and set aside.
3. In a medium saucepan over low heat, melt vegan margarine.
4. Stir in oil, yeast, black pepper, almond milk, and cheddar cheese until cheese melts and sauce becomes smooth. (Do not let the sauce scorch.)
5. Return cooked pasta to large pot.
6. Stir in cheese sauce over low heat.
7. Sprinkle paprika on top, and serve.

CHANGE IT UP: Substitute any gluten-free pasta, such as quinoa pasta, for rice pasta.

Quinoa Pasta With Mushrooms and Asparagus

Quinoa pasta picks up the rich mushroom flavor and spices of this hearty dish. Quinoa pasta is often made with rice or corn. We prefer quinoa pasta with the rice because the texture is smoother.

YIELD: 2 SERVINGS

- 8 oz. quinoa spiral pasta
- 2 c. mushrooms, sliced
- 8 oz. asparagus, trimmed and sliced into 2-inch pieces
- 1 c. fresh or frozen sweet peas
- 1 medium red onion, thinly sliced
- 3 cloves garlic, minced
- 2 T. extra-virgin olive oil
- 1 tsp. sea salt
- 1 T. chopped fresh basil (or 1 tsp. dried)

1. Prepare quinoa pasta according to package directions.
2. Drain under cold water and set aside.
3. In a large skilled cook mushrooms, asparagus, peas, onions, garlic, and oil over low heat about 5 minutes, while stirring.
4. Add quinoa pasta to vegetables and continue to cook over low heat approximately 3 minutes.
5. Stir in salt and basil, and serve warm.

Quinoa Walnut Burgers

These burgers are great alone, or placed in a gluten-free bun or lettuce leaf topped with lettuce, pickles, tomato, red onion, vegan cheddar cheese, and avocado.

Yield: 8 patties

3/4 c. water
1/2 c. uncooked quinoa
1 celery stalk, sliced
3 cloves garlic, peeled and quartered
6 scallions, sliced
1 15-oz. can black beans, drained and rinsed (or 2 c. cooked black beans)
1/2 c. walnuts, chopped
1 T. cumin
1/4 tsp. curry
1/2 tsp. sea salt
1/4 tsp. black pepper

1. Preheat oven to 350 degrees F.
2. In a small pot bring water to a boil.
3. Add quinoa, cover, and reduce heat to low.
4. Cook until liquid is absorbed, approximately 15 minutes, and set aside.
5. In a food processor, pulse celery, scallions, and garlic about 20 seconds.
6. Add cooked quinoa, beans, walnuts, cumin, curry, salt, and black pepper, and pulse until combined but still slightly chunky.
7. Form into balls and press into approximately 4-inch patties.
8. Place patties on an oiled baking sheet.
9. Reduce oven temperature to 250 degrees F.
10. Bake 10–15 minutes on each side.

Satisfying Vegetable Stew

This thick and hearty stew is delicious with gluten-free bread croutons and vegan cheese sprinkled on top.

YIELD: 4–6 SERVINGS

1 T. extra-virgin olive oil
1 large yellow onion, quartered and sliced
3 cloves garlic, minced
1 c. carrot, cut into 1/4-inch-thick slices
1 c. sliced celery
2 1/2 c. sliced mushrooms
1/2 c. water
4 medium tomatoes, diced
3 medium red potatoes, cut into 1-inch chunks (approx. 2 1/2 c.)
2 c. cooked kidney beans
1 15-oz. can tomato sauce (approx. 2 c.)
1 tsp. dried thyme
1 bay leaf
1 tsp. sea salt
1/4 tsp. curry powder
1 tsp. dried basil
3 T. oat flour

1. In large pot, heat oil.
2. Add onions, garlic, carrots, celery, and mushrooms.
3. Cook approximately 3 minutes, stirring frequently.
4. Add water, tomatoes, potatoes, beans, tomato sauce, thyme, bay leaf, sea salt, curry powder, and basil.
5. Stir 5 minutes over medium-low heat.
6. Cover, reduce heat to low, and cook 10 minutes.
7. Stir in flour and cook 5 more minutes.
8. Discard bay leaf. Serve warm.

Springtime Pasta Primavera

Primavera in Latin languages means "spring," and this dish takes advantage of spring's finest produce!

Yield: 4 servings

4 c. rice seashell pasta, cooked
1/4 c. extra-virgin olive oil
6 cloves garlic, minced
2 large carrots, biased sliced in 1/4-inch pieces
4 scallions, chopped
1 medium red bell pepper, diced in 1/2-inch pieces
10 thin asparagus stalks, sliced in 1/2-inch pieces
1/2 c. fresh basil
1 large tomato, chopped
1 T. dried Italian seasoning
1 tsp. sea salt
1 tsp. ground black pepper
1/4 c. slivered almonds

1. Place pasta in a large bowl and set aside.
2. In a large skillet cook olive oil, garlic, carrots, scallions, bell pepper, and asparagus and over low-medium heat 3 minutes stirring constantly.
3. Toss vegetables with pasta.
4. Add basil, tomatoes, Italian seasoning, sea salt, black pepper, and almonds. Stir well and serve.

CHANGE IT UP: Sprinkle 1/2 c. vegan parmesan cheese on top of pasta before serving.

Substitute pine nuts for almonds.

Sweet Potato Chili

This chili can be made with black beans or red beans. It's delicious with gluten-free cornbread.

Yield: 4 servings

4 T. extra-virgin olive oil
1 large sweet potato, peeled and diced
1 large onion, diced
1 large carrot, diced
4 cloves garlic, mined
2 T. chili powder
1 T. cumin
1 tsp. sea salt
1 c. water
2 15-oz. cans pinto beans, rinsed
1 c. chopped tomatoes
1 c. tomato sauce
1/3 c. chopped fresh cilantro
1/4 c. fresh lemon juice

1. In a large skillet cook oil, sweet potato, onion, and carrot over medium heat until onion softens but does not brown, approximately 2 minutes.
2. Add garlic, chili powder, cumin, and sea salt.
3. Continue to cook over low heat about 30 seconds, consistently stirring.
4. Add water and bring to a simmer.
5. Cover, reduce to a simmer, and cook until sweet potato is tender, approximately 15 minutes.
6. Add beans, tomatoes, tomato sauce, cilantro, and lemon juice.
7. Simmer an additional 5 minutes. Serve warm.

Tomato Spaghetti Squash With Mushrooms

Spaghetti squash is nature's spaghetti that is gluten-free and fun to make.

Yield: 2 servings

1 medium spaghetti squash
2 T. extra-virgin olive oil
1 yellow onion, chopped
3 garlic cloves, minced
1 c. sliced mushrooms
1 15-oz. can Italian tomatoes (or 2 c. chopped fresh Roma tomatoes)
1 T. chopped basil

1. Preheat oven to 350 degrees F.
2. Cut squash in half, prick holes, and scoop out seeds.
3. Fill a baking dish with water about 1/4 inch high.
4. Place squash, face up, in the dish.
5. Reduce oven temperature to 250 degrees F.
6. Bake one hour.
7. In a large skillet cook oil, onion, garlic, mushrooms, tomatoes, and basil over low heat about 8 minutes, stirring constantly.
8. When squash is tender, use a fork to remove strands from the skin.
9. Divide strands in half onto two plates.
10. Divide sauce, pouring on top of each plate of squash strands.

CHANGE IT UP: Sprinkle vegan parmesan cheese or vegan mozzarella cheese on top before serving.

Veggie Lo Mein

For this Asian-inspired dish we use a soy-free soy sauce and cut veggies to give it an authentic Asian taste. We always use alcohol- and wheat-free soy sauces, too. Soy-free soy sauce can be found at most health food stores and online. Organic rice or soba (buckwheat) works well in this recipe, and coconut soy sauce works well for the soy-free soy sauce. If you can get fresh ginger, use 1 T. minced in place of dried ginger.

YIELD: 2–4 SERVINGS

8 oz. gluten-free spaghetti
3/4 c. vegetable stock
2 T. soy-free soy sauce
1 T. maple syrup
1 T. arrowroot
1/2 tsp. red pepper flakes
1 T. extra-virgin olive oil
1/2 c. snow peas, sliced (or sugar snaps)
1/2 c. red bell pepper, thinly sliced
1 c. mung bean sprouts
6 scallions, chopped
4 cloves garlic, minced
1 T. ginger
2 T. toasted sesame seeds or hemp seeds (optional)

1. Cook pasta according to package directions.
2. Drain pasta under cold water, and set aside.
3. In a medium bowl combine broth, soy-free soy sauce, and maple syrup, and stir well.
4. Stir in arrowroot and red pepper flakes, and set aside.
5. In a large skillet cook olive oil, snow peas, red bell pepper, sprouts, and scallions over low-medium heat about 4 minutes.
6. Stir in garlic and ginger, and cook for an additional 2 minutes, stirring well.
7. Toss in pasta and stock mixture, and simmer about 4 minutes.
8. Transfer to serving platter and top with toasted sesame seeds or hemp seeds.

Veggie Sushi Supreme

Wasabi is a member of the Brassicaceae (please don't ask us to pronounce this word!) family, which includes cabbages, horseradish, and mustard. It is called Japanese horseradish, although horseradish is a different plant that is often used as a substitute for wasabi. The plant grows naturally along the stream beds in mountain river valleys of Japan. Nori sheets are made from seaweed and often called "the reservoir of vitamins" due to their high vitamin content. Nori not only has as much iron as one egg, it is an excellent source of omega-3s. If your nori rolls won't stay rolled, try "sealing" the seam with a little maple syrup. To make rolling easier and prevent the nori sheets from tearing, use an inexpensive bamboo sushi mat (available in Japanese markets and many health food stores).

YIELD: 6 SERVINGS (ROLLS)

6 c. water
3 c. short-grained brown rice
3 T. maple syrup
2/3 c. rice wine vinegar
1 medium cucumber, seeded and julienne sliced
1 small zucchini, julienne sliced
1/2 green bell pepper, seeded and julienne sliced
2 medium carrots, julienne sliced
1 package pre-toasted nori sheets (seaweed sheets)
Prepared wasabi paste

1. Bring water to a boil.
2. Add rice, lower heat, and simmer 40 minutes, stirring occasionally.
3. Cool rice and place it a large bowl.
4. Mix in maple syrup and vinegar.
5. Steam cucumber, zucchini, bell peppers, and carrots in a large pot approximately 5 minutes.
6. Let cool to room temperature.
7. Lay out the first nori sheet.
8. Place a handful of rice in the center of the sheet, moisten your hands with water, and gently but firmly press the rice to the edges of the sheet so that there is a thin layer in line on the sheet.
9. Spread a bit of wasabi paste on the top of the rice, approximately 1 1/2 inches from one edge of the nori sheet.

10. Lay vegetables strips parallel to the wasabi in a width of approximately 1 inch along the wasabi line.
11. Carefully wrap the closest edge over the vegetables, and roll the nori delicately but tightly.
12. Seal by moistening the edge of the nori.
13. Once the nori sheet is completely rolled, slice in 6 pieces and arrange on a platter.
14. Repeat with remaining nori sheets.

CHANGE IT UP: Add avocado.

Walnut Tacos With Romaine Wrap

Walnuts are loaded with omega-3s, which make them the ultimate "brain food." These incredible nuts blended with the cumin and garlic add a meaty flavor to this vegan raw taco. The Romaine lettuce leaves serve as a "taco shell," and if you want to do mini tacos then scoop the mixture into endive leaves.

YIELD: 2 SERVINGS

2 c. walnuts
1/4 tsp. cumin
1 T. balsamic vinegar
1/8 tsp. paprika
1/8 tsp. oregano
1/8 tsp. ground black pepper
1/8 tsp. garlic powder
1 T. wheat-free soy sauce or coconut "soy" sauce
2 cloves garlic, minced
6 large romaine lettuce leaves
1 Hass avocado, chopped
1/2 c. diced tomatoes
4 green onions, thinly sliced

1. Pulse walnuts, cumin, vinegar, paprika, oregano, black pepper, garlic powder, soy sauce, and garlic in a food processor about eight times, until mixture is crumbly but not over-blended.
2. Place walnut mixture evenly into the lettuces leaves.
3. Top with avocado, tomatoes, and green onions.

CHANGE IT UP: Add 6 sliced olives to each taco.

Sprinkle vegan cheddar cheese top of each taco.

Substitute a scoop of Great Guacamole on top of each taco for avocado.

Sprinkle each taco with hot sauce or salsa.

SPECTACULAR SALADS

Apple Slaw With Cranberries and Pumpkin Seeds

Avocado, Grapefruit, and Arugula Salad

Baby Spinach and Pear Salad With Hazelnuts

Black-Eyed Peas and Tomatoes With Lemon Vinaigrette

Black Rice and Mango Salad With Walnuts

Broccoli With Raisins and Slivered Almonds

Caesar Salad With Pine Nuts

Cajun Rice and Black Olive Salad

Cashew Ginger Rice Salad

Cherry Tomato and Olive Salad

Cool Coleslaw

Curried Rice Salad With Red Grapes

Dijon Almond Green Beans and Tomato Salad

Garbanzo Bean and Corn Salad

Garbanzo Beans With Fresh Basil and Walnuts

Ginger Sesame Carrot Salad

Hazelnut Green Beans in Basil Vinaigrette

Jicama Sesame Slaw

Kale Cashew Salad With Lemon Tahini Dressing

Kale Waldorf Salad

Lemon-Cilantro Chia Slaw

Mango Sesame Noodle Salad

Marinated Zucchini Salad

We love salads! Our meals are centered around a cornucopia of fresh greens and vegetables placed in a large glass bowl. Please note that whenever balsamic vinegar is used in a recipe we use "lead-free" balsamic vinegar. Whether it is naturally occurring in the soil or from the manufacturing process, lead can be present in balsamic vinegar and red wine vinegar. We prefer apple cider vinegar in our dressing and marinades. Apple cider vinegar is lead-free. You can substitute apple, red or white wine, fig, date, coconut, or apple cider vinegar in any of the recipes that call for vinegar.

Apple Slaw With Cranberries and Pumpkin Seeds

This is a colorful and tasty salad filled with antioxidants. Cranberries are known to relieve urinary tract infections. This same fruit can also help ward off ulcer and gum problems, and the combination of cranberries, apples, and pumpkin seeds makes this a memory-boosting dish.

YIELD: 6 SERVINGS

1/2 c. orange juice
1/4 c. sesame seed oil
3 T. chopped fresh cilantro
1/2 tsp. ground black pepper
1 Granny Smith apple, unpeeled, cored, and shredded
4 large carrots, grated
1 red onion, finely chopped
1/2 c. dried cranberries
1/2 c. pumpkin seeds

1. In a small bowl combine orange juice, sesame seed oil, cilantro, and black pepper.
2. In a large bowl, mix apple, carrots, and onion.
3. Stir in orange juice mixture.
4. Toss in cranberries and pumpkin seeds. Serve immediately or chill.

Avocado, Grapefruit, and Arugula Salad

Arugula is a spicy green leaf that has a peppery, mustard-y flavor. The sweet grapefruit adds a wonderful sweet flavor and avocados give the salad a perfect creamy, nutty flavor.

YIELD: 4 SERVINGS

2 T. honey
3 T. fresh lime juice
5 oz. arugula leaves
2 grapefruits, peeled, sections halved
1 avocado, diced
1/4 c. sunflower seeds, ideally soaked with water at least an hour

1. Mix honey and lime juice in a medium bowl.
2. Add arugula and mix well.
3. Toss in grapefruit sections and avocado.
4. Stir in sunflower seeds just before serving.

CHANGE IT UP: Add 1/2 c. sliced fresh strawberries or blueberries. Substitute pine nuts or flaxseeds for sunflower seeds.

Baby Spinach and Pear Salad With Hazelnuts

Spinach is such a wonderful, iron-rich green and high in vitamin K, which is great for the brain! Bosc pears adds a burst of sweetness.

YIELDS: 4–6 SERVINGS

8 c. lightly packed fresh baby spinach leaves, lightly stemmed
2 firm but ripe Bosc pears, unpeeled, quartered lengthwise, cored, and cut
1 c. red onion, thinly sliced
1/2 c. raisins
2/3 c. hazelnuts, chopped
1/2 c. extra-virgin olive oil
3 T. balsamic vinegar
2 tsp. whole-grain mustard
1 T. raw honey
1/2 tsp. kosher sea salt
1/2 tsp. ground black pepper

1. Place spinach, pears, onions, raisins, and hazelnuts in a large bowl.
2. In a jar, mix oil, vinegar, mustard, honey, salt, and pepper well.
3. Pour dressing over spinach mixture.

Black-Eyed Peas and Tomatoes With Lemon Vinaigrette

This Middle Eastern–type dish is packed with protein and fiber.

YIELD: 6 SERVINGS

1/4 c. lemon juice
2 cloves garlic, minced
1 tsp. Dijon mustard
1/2 tsp. sea salt
1/4 tsp. ground black pepper
1/4 c. extra-virgin olive oil
2 15-oz. cans black eyed peas, rinsed and drained
1 medium red onion, quartered and thinly sliced
1 c. cherry or grape tomatoes, halved
1/2 c. coarsely chopped parsley
1/4 c. parsley sprigs, for garnish

1. In a medium bowl, combine lemon juice, garlic, Dijon mustard, salt, and pepper.
2. Whisk in olive oil until completely emulsified.
3. Stir in black-eyed peas, red onion, tomatoes, and parsley.
4. Refrigerate at least 1 hour, and serve garnished with parsley springs.

Black Rice and Mango Salad With Walnuts

Mangos and raisins give an added sweet twist to this salad. Mangos are filled with antioxidants, which is terrific for brain health. Black rice is an heirloom variety of rice cultivated in Asia, and it is an excellent source of fiber.

YIELD: 2 SERVINGS

1 c. black rice
2 c. water
2 c. diced mango
1/2 c. thinly sliced green onion
1/4 c. finely chopped parsley
2 T. finely chopped cilantro
2 T. finely chopped mint
1/4 c. extra-virgin olive oil
1/2 c. raisins
1/3 c. chopped walnuts

1. In a large saucepan bring water to a boil.
2. Add rice to water.
3. Reduce heat to a simmer.
4. Cook rice 35 minutes or until tender.
5. Drain rice and cool.
6. Transfer rice to a large bowl.
7. Stir in mango, green onions, parsley, cilantro, and mint.
8. Drizzle olive oil around the mixture and stir.
9. Toss with raisins and walnuts. Serve fresh or chilled.

Broccoli With Raisins and Slivered Almonds

Broccoli is filled with powerful antioxidants. Rice vinegar, honey, and raisins add a sweet flavor that is perfect with almonds. This can be served immediately or stored in the refrigerator for up to four days.

YIELD: 4 SERVINGS

1/3 c. rice vinegar
1/3 c. extra-virgin olive oil
3 T. honey
1 tsp. sea salt
1/2 tsp. ground black pepper
12 c. broccoli florets (from 2 large bunches), raw or steamed
1/2 c. raisins
1/4 c. slivered almonds

1. In a medium bowl whisk together vinegar, olive oil, honey, sea salt, and black pepper.
2. Place broccoli florets in a medium bowl.
3. Pour olive oil and vinegar mixture on top of broccoli and mix well.
4. Stir in raisins and almonds.

Caesar Salad With Pine Nuts

This vegan Caesar salad is filled with flavor. The traditional anchovy paste used in many Caesar salads is not missed in this tasty dish!

Yield: 2 servings

1 head romaine lettuce
1 red tomato, chopped
1/4 c. extra-virgin olive oil
2 T. fresh lemon juice
2 cloves garlic, minced
1/2 tsp. sea salt
1/4 tsp. ground black pepper
1/4 c. gluten-free croutons
1/4 c. grated vegan parmesan or mozzarella cheese, optional
1/4 c. pine nuts

1. Break lettuce into bite-sized pieces and place in large bowl.
2. Add tomato.
3. In a separate small bowl whisk olive oil, lemon juice, garlic, salt, and black pepper.
4. Place croutons and vegan cheese on top of salad.
5. Pour dressing on top and toss well.
6. Sprinkle with pine nuts and serve immediately.

Cajun Rice and Black Olive Salad

This Cajun salad is a seasoned and spicy salad bursting with flavor. It can be stored in refrigerator for up to five days.

YIELD: 2–4 SERVINGS

2 T. extra-virgin olive oil
2 T. apple cider vinegar
1 tsp. dried marjoram leaves
1 tsp. dried thyme leaves
2 cloves garlic, minced
1 tsp. hot sauce
2 large red tomatoes, diced
1 c. sliced black olives
2 c. cooked brown rice
1 15-oz. can kidney beans, well drained
6 green onions, thinly sliced
1 large celery stalk, diced

1. In a large bowl mix olive oil, vinegar, marjoram, thyme, garlic, and hot sauce.
2. Stir in tomatoes, black olives, rice, beans, green onions, and celery.
3. Serve immediately or serve chilled.

Cashew Ginger Rice Salad

Cashews, lime, and fresh ginger give this salad a sweet, spicy flavor.

YIELD: 2–4 SERVINGS

Dressing:

2 T. freshly grated ginger
1/2 c. freshly squeezed lime juice
1/4 c. extra-virgin olive oil
3 cloves garlic, minced
1/4 tsp. sea salt
1/4 tsp. ground black pepper

Salad:

2 c. cooked brown rice
1 red bell pepper, seeded and chopped finely
1 c. cubed tempeh
4 scallions, chopped finely
1/2 c. chopped cashews

1. Whisk together grated ginger, lime juice , olive oil, garlic, salt, and black pepper, and set aside.
2. Combine cooked rice, bell pepper, tempeh, and scallions in a large bowl.
3. Add dressing, and toss until well combined.
4. Garnish with cashews.

Cherry Tomato and Olive Salad

Cherry tomatoes are wonderful to use in salads because they are sweet and colorful. Toasted sunflower seeds add a wonderful crunch to this refreshing salad.

YIELD: 4 SERVINGS

40 cherry tomatoes, halved
1 c. pitted, sliced black olives
6 green onions, thinly sliced
1/2 c. extra-virgin olive oil
1/3 c. red wine vinegar
2 T. fresh basil, chopped (or 1 T. dried, but fresh is preferred)
1/4 tsp. sea salt
2 cloves garlic, minced

1. Place tomatoes, olives, and green onions in a medium bowl.
2. In a small bowl whisk olive oil, red wine vinegar, basil, sea salt, and minced garlic.
3. Stir in olive oil mixture to tomatoes, olives, and onions. Serve immediately or serve chilled

CHANGE IT UP: Add 1/2 c. flaxseeds (for extra crunch and a dose of omega-3s!).

Cool Coleslaw

Follow Your Heart's Low-Fat Veganaise (soy-free version) adds a creamy, delicious flavor to the coleslaw. However, you can use a vegan mayonnaise of your choice or make your own. We like to add cabbage to as many dishes as we can because it is a terrific blood detoxifier and brain-boosting food! Cabbage is loaded with vitamin C, sulfur, and iodine, which is excellent for the brain. The longer the coleslaw marinates, the richer the flavor. The coleslaw will last up to a week in the refrigerator.

YIELD: 6 C.

2 c. shredded green cabbage
2 c. shredded purple cabbage
1 c. grated carrots
1 medium yellow onion, chopped
4 green onions, sliced
3/4 c. Veganaise
1/2 c. fresh lemon juice
3 T. pure maple syrup
1 tsp. ground black pepper

1. Place green cabbage, purple cabbage, carrots, and onions into a large mixing bowl.
2. Add Veganaise and mix well.
3. Add lemon juice, maple syrup, and black pepper.
4. Refrigerate in an airtight bowl at least 3 hours, and serve.

CHANGE IT UP: Add 1/2 c. corn kernels and 1/2 c. nuts.

During the holidays, add 1/2 c. fresh or dried cranberries.

Curried Rice Salad With Red Grapes

Curry mixed with grapes and raisins makes this rice a spicy, sweet delight!

YIELD: 2 SERVINGS

2 c. brown rice, cooked
1/2 c. diced celery
1/2 c. raisins
1 c. seedless red grapes, halved
1/2 c. sliced green onions
1/4 c. extra-virgin olive oil
1/4 c. lemon juice
1 T. curry powder
1/4 tsp. ground black pepper

1. In a large bowl mix rice, celery, raisins, grapes, and green onions.
2. In a small bowl whisk olive oil, lemon juice, curry powder, and pepper.
3. Stir olive oil dressing into rice mixture. Serve fresh or chilled.

Dijon Almond Green Beans and Tomato Salad

We enjoy eating green beans raw and steamed. Sweet cherry tomatoes and red onion add a delicious flavor to these green beans.

YIELD: 4–6 SERVINGS

2 lb. green string beans
1 1/2 tsp. Dijon mustard
2 T. red wine vinegar
1/4 c. plus 1 T. extra-virgin olive oil
1/2 tsp. sea salt
1 T. chopped tarragon
1 T. chopped chives
1/2 tsp. dried thyme
1 medium red onion, thinly sliced
1/2 lb. cherry tomatoes, halved
1/2 c. slivered almonds

1. Steam green beans until crisp-tender, about 4 minutes.
2. Drain and rinse green beans under cold water until chilled, and pat dry.
3. In a large bowl whisk mustard with vinegar.
4. Whisk in olive oil and sea salt.
5. Add green beans, tarragon, chives, and thyme, and toss to coat.
6. Gently toss in tomatoes, red onions, and almonds, and serve.

Garbanzo Bean and Corn Salad

Garbanzo beans (chickpeas) are high in magnesium and dietary fiber, which are both great for the brain, and help with digestion and blood circulation! Red onion and fresh corn bring a sweet flavor to this delicious dish! For the sake of time we use canned garbanzo beans, but you can soak and cook garbanzo beans fresh.

YIELD: 2 SERVINGS

1 15-oz. can chickpeas, drained and rinsed (or 2 c. fresh cooked)
2/3 c. steamed corn kernels
1/4 c. diced cucumber
1 small red onion, diced
1/4 c. diced red bell pepper
2 garlic cloves, minced
1 large tomato, diced
2 T. fresh parsley, finely chopped
4 T. extra-virgin olive oil
4 T. lemon juice
1/4 tsp. sea salt
1/4 tsp. ground black pepper

1. Place chickpeas, corn, cucumber, red onion, bell pepper, garlic, tomato, and parsley in a medium bowl.
2. Whisk together olive oil, lemon juice, sea salt, and pepper.
3. Toss dressing over chickpea mixture, and refrigerate for at least an hour.

Garbanzo Beans With Fresh Basil and Walnuts

Garbanzo beans, also known as chickpeas, are often used in Mediterranean dishes. This dish can be served fresh or chilled.

YIELD: 2 SERVINGS

1 15-oz. can chickpeas, drained and rinsed
1 large tomato, diced
1/2 c. diced celery
1/2 c. chopped basil leaves
3 cloves garlic, minced
6 green onions, thinly sliced
3 T. apple cider vinegar
3 T. extra-virgin olive oil
1 tsp. dried parsley
1/4 tsp. ground black pepper
1/4 tsp. sea salt
1/2 c. walnut pieces

1. Place garbanzo beans, tomato, celery, basil, garlic, and green onion in a large bowl.
2. Mix in apple cider vinegar, olive oil, parsley, black pepper, and sea salt.
3. Serve salad fresh, or refrigerate chickpea mixture in an airtight container at least 1 hour for the flavors to marinate. Stir in walnuts before serving.

Ginger Sesame Carrot Salad

Sesame seeds and ginger give a light crunch to this classic carrot salad.

YIELD: 2 SERVINGS

1/4 c. toasted sesame seed oil
2 T. rice vinegar
2 T. sesame seed butter (tahini)
1 T. grated, fresh ginger
1/2 tsp. ground black pepper
4 large carrots, grated
2 T. chopped fresh parsley
2 T. sesame seeds

1. In a small bowl whisk together sesame seed oil, rice vinegar, sesame seed butter, ginger, and pepper.
2. Place carrots in a medium bowl.
3. Stir in sesame rice vinegar dressing.
4. Stir in parsley and sesame seeds. Serve immediately or serve chilled.

CHANGE IT UP: Add 1/2 c. raisins.

Hazelnut Green Beans in Basil Vinaigrette

Green beans can be steamed or eaten raw. Using raw green beans, scallions, and hazelnuts gives this salad a wonderful crunchy flavor. This salad can be refrigerated for up to five days.

YIELD: 4 SERVINGS

1 lb. fresh green beans, chopped
6 scallions, finely chopped
1 cucumber, diced
1 small red bell pepper, diced
1/3 c. apple cider vinegar
1/3 c. extra-virgin olive oil
2 garlic cloves, minced
1 tsp. dried basil
1/2 tsp. sea salt
1/2 tsp. ground black pepper
1/4 c. hazelnuts (filberts)

1. In large bowl, place green beans, green onions, cucumber, and red bell pepper.
2. In small bowl whisk vinegar, olive oil, minced garlic, basil, sea salt, and black pepper.
3. Stir olive oil and vinegar mixture into green bean mixture.
4. Chill 1 hour, add hazelnuts, and serve.

Jicama Sesame Slaw

This jicama-infused slaw makes a wonderful light snack or side dish.

YIELD: 1–2 SERVINGS

2 c. grated jicama
1/2 c. grated red onion
2 T. sesame seed oil
1 T. honey
1/4 c. lime juice
2 T. sesame seeds

1. In medium bowl mix jicama and onion.
2. In small bowl mix sesame seed oil, honey, and lime juice.
3. Stir sesame seed oil mixture into jicama and red onions.
4. Sprinkle sesame seeds on top and serve, or serve chilled.

Kale Cashew Salad With Lemon Tahini Dressing

We use soy-free soy sauce such as coconut aminos, which is a soy-free sauce that is wheat-free, too. This dressing is also excellent on a bed of lettuce or served as a dip for cucumbers, carrots, bell peppers, and celery. We like to smother this tasty dressing all over the salad, but you might want less. Any extra dressing can be stored for a week in the refrigerator; it tastes great on all green salads or steamed vegetables.

YIELD: 4 SERVINGS

Salad:

4 c. chopped raw kale (about 1/2 small bunch)
1 c. grated carrots
1 avocado, diced
1 small red onion, diced
1 celery stalk, diced
1/2 c. cashews

Dressing:

3/4 c. tahini (toasted sesame seed butter)
1/3 c. fresh lemon juice
1/4 c. soy-free soy sauce
1/2 c. extra-virgin olive oil
1/4 c. chopped green bell pepper
1 stalk celery, chopped
1 medium yellow onion, chopped
3 cloves garlic, skinned and cut in quarters

1. Place kale, carrots, avocado, red onion, celery, and cashews in a large bowl and set aside.
2. In a blender or food processor, blend tahini, lemon juice, and soy-free soy sauce 15 seconds.
3. Add bell pepper, celery, onion, and garlic to tahini mixture and blend until smooth.
4. Pour half of the dressing at a time onto salad to reach your desired amount.

Kale Waldorf Salad

Kale adds extra brain boosting phytonutrients to this classic Waldorf salad. Fuji apples are best, but any kind will work.

YIELD: 2–4 SERVINGS

Salad:

3 c. chopped kale
1 c. grated apple
1 red onion, diced
1 c. diced celery
3/4 c. chopped walnuts

Dressing:

1/4 c. sunflower seeds
1/4 c. cashews
1/4 c. water
1/2 c. lemon juice
1 tsp. mustard
2 garlic cloves, minced
2 T. extra-virgin olive oil
1/2 tsp. sea salt
1/4 tsp. black pepper

1. In a large bowl place kale, shredded apples, red onion, celery, and walnuts.
2. Blend sunflower seeds, cashews, lemon juice, mustard, garlic, oil, sea salt, and pepper in a food processor until smooth.
3. Pour dressing over salad and mix well.

Lemon-Cilantro Chia Slaw

This coleslaw is a light alternative to the traditional mayonnaise- and sugar-laced coleslaw. This tasty salad can be stored in the refrigerator for up to a week.

YIELD: 2–4 SERVINGS

1 green cabbage, thinly sliced
1 large yellow onion, grated
2 large carrots, grated
1/4 c. chia seeds
1/4 c. lemon juice
2 T. maple syrup
1 T. fresh cilantro, finely diced
1 T. Dijon mustard
2/3 c. extra-virgin olive oil

1. Place cabbage, onions, carrots, and chia seeds in a large bowl.
2. In a blender, blend lemon juice, maple syrup, cilantro, and mustard 10 seconds.
3. While blender is on, slowly add olive oil and blend until smooth.
4. Pour dressing over cabbage mixture, and mix well.
5. Chill and serve.

Mango Sesame Noodle Salad

Mango gives a sweet twist to this delicious salad.

YIELD: 4–6 SERVINGS

12 oz. soba noodles
4 T. extra-virgin olive oil
3 T. rice vinegar
3 T. lemon juice
3 T. honey
1/4 tsp. cayenne pepper
1/2 tsp. sea salt
4 green onions, thinly sliced
1/4 c. diced celery
2 carrots, grated
2 mangos, peeled and diced
1/4 c. chopped cilantro
2 T. sesame seeds

1. In a large pot, boil noodles until tender but firm to bite, about 8 minutes.
2. Drain and rinse noodles under running cold water.
3. Transfer noodles a large bowl.
4. In a separate large bowl combine oil, vinegar, lemon juice, honey, cayenne pepper, and salt, using a whisk or a long-tooth fork to mix well.
5. Add noodles, green onions, celery, carrots, mango, and cilantro, and toss.
6. Refrigerate at least two hours, stirring salad every half hour to make sure noodles absorb dressing evenly.
7. Serve salad cold, tossed with the sesame seeds

Marinated Zucchini Salad

This dish picks up the flavors best when it marinades for at least four hours.

YIELD: 4 SERVINGS

1/4 c. lemon juice
1 clove garlic, minced
1 tsp. sea salt
1/8 tsp. black pepper
3 T. extra-virgin olive oil
1 lb. medium zucchini, thinly sliced
1 T. parsley, finely chopped
1 T. mint, finely chopped
1 tsp. dill

1. Mix lemon juice, garlic, sea salt, black pepper, and olive oil.
2. Toss with the zucchini.
3. Refrigerate at least four hours.
4. Add parsley, mint, and dill to marinated zucchini, and stir gently. Serve immediately.

CHANGE IT UP: Adding 1/2 c. diced red bell pepper and 1/2 c. pine nuts for a sweet, nutty flavor.

Mixed Berry Salad With Pecans

This very berry salad topped with a sweet-tart dressing and pine nuts make an ideal midday snack.

YIELD: 4 SERVINGS

2 c. strawberries, tops cut off
1 c. blueberries
1 c. raspberries
1/2 c. blackberries
2 T. balsamic vinegar
2 T. maple syrup
1/2 c. pecans

1. Place strawberries, blueberries, raspberries, and blackberries in a large bowl.
2. In small bowl whisk together balsamic vinegar and maple syrup.
3. Pour vinegar-syrup mixture over berries.
4. Top with pecans and serve.

CHANGE IT UP: Substitute 1/2 c. Cashew Coconut Granola (page 177) for pecans.

Moroccan Beet Salad

This is a chilled salad that tastes great alone, on top of a bed of quinoa, or over mixed greens.

YIELD: 2–4 SERVINGS

4 large beets
1 medium red onion, thinly sliced
2/3 c. pecan pieces
3 T. lemon juice
2 cloves garlic, minced
3/4 tsp. cumin
1/4 tsp. sea salt
1/8 tsp. black pepper
6 T. extra-virgin olive oil

1. Steam beets over medium heat 45 minutes or until tender when pierced with a fork.
2. Cool, peel, and cut beets into bite-sized pieces (diced).
3. Place beets, red onions, and pecans in a medium bowl.
4. In a small bowl whisk lemon juice, garlic, cumin, sea salt, pepper, and olive oil.
5. Pour dressing over beet mixture and chill for a couple hours.

Napa Cilantro Slaw

Napa cabbage is known as "Chinese cabbage," as it originated near Beijing, China, and is widely used in East Asian cuisine. Napa cabbage, in comparison to green or red cabbage, is a tad milder and sweeter, making it a perfect fit for this refreshing slaw. This slaw can also be made with savoy cabbage. When marinated this salad has a consistency and flavor of a combination between a traditional coleslaw and sauerkraut. This will keep a week in the refrigerator.

YIELD: 4–6 SERVINGS

Slaw:

3 c. shredded Napa cabbage
1 c. shredded red cabbage
1 c. grated carrots
3/4 c. grated golden beet
4 green onions, sliced (approx. 1/4 c.)
3 T. chopped fresh cilantro
1/2 tsp. ground black pepper
1 tsp. sea salt
3 T. sesame seeds (optional)

Dressing:

2 T. miso
4 T. apple juice
2 T. toasted sesame seed oil
2 T. apple cider vinegar
2 cloves garlic, minced

1. Place Napa cabbage, red cabbage, carrots, beets, green onion, and cilantro in a large bowl.
2. In a separate small bowl whisk (or use a fork to stir) miso, apple juice, toasted sesame seed oil, vinegar, and garlic until mixed well.
3. Add dressing to cabbage mixture and stir well.
4. Stir in pepper, sea salt, and sesame seeds. Served or marinate overnight.

CHANGE IT UP: Substitute 1/2 c. peanuts, almonds, or cashews for sesame seeds.

Penne Pine Nut Pasta Salad

Preparing this salad the night before you eat it is worth it! On a hot summer day it's great to pull this salad out of the refrigerator, and toss it over a bed of greens or eat it right out of the bowl.

YIELD: 2 SERVINGS

8 oz. rice penne pasta
1/3 c. apple cider vinegar
1/4 c. extra virgin oil
1/2 c. sliced black olives
8 oz. cherry tomatoes, halved (about 1 c.)
1/2 c. shelled fresh peas
2 cloves garlic, minced
2 tsp. dried basil
1 tsp. sea salt
1 tsp. freshly ground black pepper
1/2 c. pine nuts

1. Cook pasta according to the package directions.
2. Drain pasta and transfer to a large bowl.
3. Stir in vinegar and olive oil.
4. Mix in olives, peas, garlic, basil, sea salt, and black pepper.
5. Refrigerate in a covered bowl at least two hours or overnight.
6. Stir in pine nuts just before serving.

Persian Rice With Pistachios

Basmati rice has a fluffy texture that is ideal for this sweet and savory salad. This can be eaten warm or cold, and it will last in the refrigerator for up to a week.

Yield: 2 servings

2 c. cooked brown basmati rice, cooled
1 tsp. saffron
1/2 tsp. sea salt
1/8 tsp. turmeric
1/8 tsp. red pepper flakes
1/2 c. grated carrots
1/3 c. diced red bell pepper
1/4 c. raisins
1/2 c. pistachios
1 T. lemon juice

1. In a large bowl mix well basmati rice, saffron, sea salt, turmeric, and red pepper flakes.
2. Stir in carrots, red bell pepper, raisins, pistachios, and lemon juice.

Quinoa Tabouli Salad

This salad is traditionally made with bulgur, a form of wheat. Quinoa (pronounced KEEN-wha), is 100-percent whole grain that is certified gluten-free, and is a complete source of protein, low in the glycemic index, and high in amino acids. Quinoa is a versatile grain that picks up flavors nicely. With quinoa, you won't miss the bulgur, and you'll enjoy the delicious flavors of the fresh herbs. Follow the cooking instructions on the quinoa package.

Yield: 2 servings

1 c. cooked quinoa
3 medium red tomatoes, diced
1/4 c. minced fresh parsley
1/4 c. minced fresh mint
1 medium cucumber, peeled and diced
4 cloves garlic, minced
1 small red onion, diced
4 T. extra-virgin olive oil
4 T. lemon juice

1. In medium bowl mix quinoa, tomatoes, parsley, mint, cucumber, garlic, and onion.
2. Stir in oil and lemon juice.
3. Refrigerate for at least 1 hour. Serve chilled.

Radicchio Quinoa Salad With Nectarines and Walnuts

Radicchio is a rich source of fiber, vitamins, and minerals! It has high amounts of antioxidants and plant phytonutrients, and is an excellent source of vitamin K, which helps limit neuronal damage to the brain. Sweet nectarines offset the slight bitterness of radicchio.

YIELD: 2 SERVINGS

4 T. extra-virgin olive oil
2 T. apple cider vinegar
1/2 tsp. Dijon mustard
1/2 tsp. sea salt
1/4 tsp. black pepper
2 c. cooked quinoa, cooled
2 large, firm, ripe nectarines, diced
1 head radicchio, coarsely chopped
1/2 c. walnuts

1. In a small bowl, whisk together oil, vinegar, and mustard.
2. Stir in salt and pepper.
3. In a large bowl, combine quinoa, nectarines, and radicchio.
4. Add dressing and gently toss to coat salad.
5. Sprinkle walnuts on top and serve.

CHANGE IT UP: Substitute peaches for nectarines.
Add 1/2 c. raisins.

Red Kidney Bean Salad With Papaya and Cilantro

This salad is delicious served alone or on top of a bed of romaine lettuce.

YIELD: 2–4 SERVINGS

2 T. finely minced fresh ginger
1/2 c. rice wine vinegar
2 T. sesame oil
1/2 tsp. black pepper
1 c. kidney beans
1 c. diced fresh papaya
1 c. coarsely chopped fresh cilantro
1 Hass avocado, sliced
1/4 c. flaxseeds

1. In a medium bowl, mix ginger, rice vinegar, sesame oil, and black pepper.
2. Add kidney beans, papaya, and cilantro.

3. Place the salad in the refrigerator for at least 20 minutes to let the flavors marinate.
4. Top with avocado and flaxseeds.

CHANGE IT UP: Add 1/2 c. cubed fresh mango.
Substitute garbanzo beans for kidney beans.

Shredded Cabbage With Orange Vinaigrette

Red and white cabbage combined with red bell peppers and carrots makes this a colorful salad. The dressing adds just the right amount of sweetness to this salad.

YIELD: 4 SERVINGS

Salad:

2 c. shredded white cabbage
1 c. shredded red cabbage
1/4 c. diced red bell pepper
1 1/2 c. shredded carrots
1/4 c. raisins

Dressing:

2 1/2 cup orange juice (approximately the juice of 4 oranges)
3/4 c. extra-virgin olive oil
1 T. Dijon mustard
1 T. fresh minced ginger
1 tsp. ground black pepper

1. In a large bowl mix cabbages, bell pepper, carrots, and raisins.
2. In separate bowl whisk together orange juice, olive oil, mustard, ginger, and black pepper.
3. Pour dressing over cabbage mixture, and toss.
4. Marinate at least 1 hour in the refrigerator before serving.

Southwest Black Bean Salad

Cilantro and corn give the perfect spice and sweetness to this black bean salad.

YIELD: 2–4 SERVINGS

2 c. cooked corn kernels
1 15-oz. can black beans, rinsed
1/2 c. sliced black olives
2 green onions, sliced
1 red onion, diced
1 tomato, diced
1 c. shredded red cabbage
1/4 c. lime juice
1/4 c. extra-virgin olive oil
1/4 c. chopped fresh cilantro
1/2 tsp. sea salt
1/8 tsp. ground black pepper

1. In medium bowl place corn, beans, olives, green onions, red onion, tomato, and cabbage.
2. In small bowl whisk lime juice, olive oil, cilantro, sea salt, and pepper.
3. Pour dressing over bean mixture, and stir until well coated. Serve immediately or chill.

CHANGE IT UP: Add 1/2 c. sunflower seeds and 1 diced ripe avocado. Add a heaping tablespoon Great Guacamole.

Spanish Rice and Corn Salad

Red bell pepper gives a sweet, crunchy flavor to this Spanish rice salad.

YIELD: 2–4 SERVINGS

2 c. cooked brown rice
1 medium tomato, diced
1 red onion, diced
1 red bell pepper, seeded and diced
1/2 c. cooked corn kernels
1 celery stalk, finely chopped
1 avocado, diced
2 T. finely chopped cilantro
4 T. extra-virgin olive oil
4 T. lemon juice
1 tsp. sea salt
1/2 tsp. chili powder
1/8 tsp. red pepper flakes
3 cloves garlic, minced

1. In a large bowl mix brown rice, tomato, onion, bell pepper, corn, celery, avocado, and cilantro.
2. In a small bowl whisk olive oil, lemon juice, sea salt, chili powder, red pepper flakes, and minced garlic.
3. Stir dressing into rice mixture. Serve immediately or chilled.

CHANGE IT UP: Add 1/2 c. black beans and 1/2 c. sliced black olives.

Super Sprout Salad

We sprout our own sprouts. It's easy, and sprouts are filled with protein and nutrients that are great for the brain!

YIELD: 4 SERVINGS

Salad:

1 c. cabbage, finely grated
1/2 c. lentil sprouts
1/2 c. alfalfa or clover sprouts
2 c. grated carrot
1/2 c. red bell pepper, diced
1/3 c. raw sunflower seeds, soaked

Dressing:

3 T. lemon juice
3 T. raw sesame seed butter (tahini)
2 T. gluten-free soy sauce (tamari)
1 T. nutritional yeast

1. Place cabbage, sprouts, carrot, bell pepper, and sunflower seeds in a medium bowl.
2. Blend lemon juice, sesame seed butter, soy sauce, and nutritional yeast well.
3. Stir dressing into vegetable and sprout mixture, and serve or chill 1 hour and then serve.

CHANGE IT UP: Add sunflower seed sprouts.

Substitute sunflower seed sprouts for lentil or alfalfa sprouts.

Thai Cucumber Salad With Peanut Chili Vinaigrette

Cucumber skins can be kept on or taken off in this wonderful salad. This salad tastes great served right away or chilled.

YIELD: 2 SERVINGS

Salad:

2 large cucumbers, chopped
6 green onions, sliced
1 c. diced red bell pepper
1 c. grated carrots
1/4 c. chopped cilantro
2 cloves garlic, minced

Dressing:

2 T. lime juice
1 T. honey
2 T. peanut butter
3 T. gluten-free soy sauce
1/4 tsp. black pepper
1/2 tsp. red pepper flakes
2 T. rice vinegar
1 T. sesame oil
2 T. water
1/2 c. dry roasted peanuts

1. Place cucumber, green onions, bell pepper, carrots, cilantro, and garlic in a medium bowl, and set aside.
2. Blend lime juice, honey, peanut butter, soy sauce, pepper flakes, vinegar, oil, and water in a blender until smooth.
3. Stir dressing and peanuts into cucumber mixture. Serve immediately or serve chilled.

SUPER SOUPS

Avocado Gazpacho
Berry Soup
Broccoli Pine Nut Soup
Broccoli Potato Cheese Soup
Butternut Squash Soup
Cajun Vegetable Gumbo
Cannellini and Pasta Soup
Carrot Bisque Soup
Cauliflower Curry Soup
Cauliflower Potato Soup
Chilled Cucumber Grape Soup
Classic Vegetable Stock
Corn Cashew Chowder
Cream of Mushroom Soup
Creamy Tomato Basil Soup

Avocado Gazpacho

Avocados are at their peak during the summertime, and this is a refreshing soup.

YIELD: 4 SERVINGS

2 c. water
3 large ripe Hass avocados, chopped
1 large cucumber, cubed
3/4 c. fresh chopped cilantro
3 garlic cloves, minced
1 small red onion, chopped
3 T. fresh lime juice
1 T. avocado oil
1 tsp. sea salt
1/2 tsp. cumin
1/4 tsp. black pepper
2/2 c. sliced green onions, for garnish
1/2 c. diced tomatoes, for garnish
1/2 c. diced avocados, for garnish
1 T. chopped cilantro, for garnish

1. Puree water, avocados, cucumber, cilantro, garlic, red onion, lime juice, avocado oil, sea salt, cumin, and black pepper in a blender until smooth.
2. Chill at least 3 hours.
3. In a small bowl gently combine green onions, tomatoes, avocado, and cilantro, and use to garnish each serving.

Berry Soup

Berry season is at its peak during the summer months. Fresh berries create a sweet and satisfying summer soup.

YIELD: 2 SERVINGS

2 1/2 c. fresh berries (blueberries, blackberries, raspberries, strawberries; or 1 16-oz. bag frozen berries)
2 c. apple juice
3 6-inch cinnamon sticks
2 whole cloves
2 T. arrowroot flour
1 tsp. extract

1. Place berries in a large saucepan.
2. Add 1 3/4 c. apple juice, cinnamon sticks, and cloves, and bring to a boil.
3. Reduce heat to a simmer and simmer approximately 8 minutes.
4. Add remaining apple juice to mixture.
5. Stir arrowroot and continue to cook until mixture begins to slightly thicken, approximately 2 more minutes.
6. Remove from heat and stir in vanilla.
7. Discard the cinnamon stick and whole cloves. Serve warm or chilled.

Broccoli Pine Nut Soup

Toasted pine nuts add a nutty flavor to this creamy soup.

Yield: 4–6 servings

1 large yellow onion, chopped
3 cloves garlic, peeled and cut in quarters
2 1/2 lb. broccoli, trimmed and cut into florets
1/2 c. pine nuts
5 1/2 c. vegetable stock
1 tsp. rosemary
1 tsp. thyme
1 T. basil
1 tsp. sea salt
2 T. pine nuts, for garnish

1. Cook onions, garlic, broccoli, and vegetable stock in a large, covered pot over medium-low heat 20 minutes.
2. Remove from heat and stir in 1/2 c. pine nuts, rosemary, thyme, basil, and sea salt.
3. Blend all ingredients in a food processor or blender, in batches, until smooth.
4. Return soup to pan and heat about 8 minutes and serve warm, garnished with pine nuts.

Broccoli Potato Cheese Soup

Adding a vegan cheese to this soup gives it a creamy texture with a cheese-like flavor.

Yield: 4 servings

1 1/2 c. fresh broccoli florets
1 medium yellow onion, diced
1 T. extra-virgin olive oil
3 cloves garlic, minced
3 c. vegetable stock
2 c. diced russet potatoes
1/2 tsp. sea salt
1/4 tsp. ground nutmeg
1 c. almond milk
1 c. shredded vegan cheddar cheese

1. Steam broccoli florets and onions about 5 minutes.
2. Bring broccoli, onions, oil, garlic, vegetable stock, potatoes, sea salt, and nutmeg to a boil in a large, covered pot.
3. Reduce the heat to low and simmer about 20 minutes, or until potatoes are tender.
4. Stir in almond milk and vegan cheese, and simmer another 5 minutes. Serve hot.

Butternut Squash Soup

Pears and butternut squash give this soup a delicate, sweet flavor.

YIELD: 4 SERVINGS

2 medium leeks, white and tender green parts finely chopped (3 c.)
1 medium butternut squash, peeled and cut into 1-inch pieces (2 lb.)
3 T. extra-virgin olive oil
3 Bartlett pears, peeled, cored and cut into 1-inch pieces (1 1/2 lb.)
5 c. vegetable stock
1 14-oz. can coconut milk
1 tsp. thyme
1 tsp. rosemary
1 T. chopped fresh basil
1/2 tsp. sea salt
1 tsp. oregano

1. Steam leeks and squash about 10 minutes.
2. In a large pot bring vegetable stock, leeks, squash, oil, and pears to a boil.
3. Reduce heat to a simmer and cook until squash is tender, approximately 35 minutes.
4. Stir in coconut milk.
5. Let cool and then blend mixture in a food processor or blender until smooth.
6. Return mixture to large pot and add thyme, rosemary, basil, sea salt, and oregano.
7. Stir over low heat about 5 minutes. Serve warm.

Cajun Vegetable Gumbo

When gumbo was first made in the 18th century, it was referred to as a dish containing stewed okra. In this recipe we added the rice to the gumbo, but you can cook the soup and pour it over a bed of seasoned cooked brown rice, too.

YIELD: 4–6 SERVINGS

2 lb. greens (collard, mustard, or turnip), washed and stemmed
1/3 c. extra-virgin olive oil
2 large yellow onions, finely diced
1 green bell pepper, finely diced
4 stalks celery, finely diced
1 16-oz. can plum tomatoes, drained and coarsely chopped
6 c. vegetable stock
1/4 c. oat flour
1 tsp. chili pepper
1 tsp. cumin
1 tsp. thyme
1 tsp. basil
1/2 tsp. oregano
1/4 c. fresh parsley, chopped
3 garlic cloves, minced
1 10-oz. package frozen okra
1 16-oz. can kidney beans, drained and rinsed
2 c. cooked brown rice

1. In a large pot place greens with enough water to just cover them and bring to a boil.
2. Reduce heat to a simmer and cook approximately 15 minutes.
3. Drain, reserving the cooked water.
4. Coarsely chop the greens and set aside.
5. In a large soup pot, over low heat, stir olive oil, onions, bell pepper, celery, and tomatoes about 5 minutes.
6. Stir in vegetable stock and greens, and continually stir over low-medium heat about 5 minutes.
7. Stir in oat flour, chili powder, cumin, thyme, basil, oregano, parsley, garlic, okra, kidney beans, and rice.
8. Simmer 10 minutes and serve warm.

Cannellini and Pasta Soup

Cannellini beans, with their mild flavor, give this soup a creamy texture. These white, fiber-rich beans are loaded with antioxidants that help prevent dementia.

YIELD: 6 SERVINGS

1 medium-sized fennel bulb, finely chopped (1 c.)
1 medium yellow onion, chopped (1 c.)
2 stalks celery, chopped
1 T. extra-virgin olive oil
3 cloves garlic, chopped
1 tsp. dried oregano
1/4 tsp. red pepper flakes
1 T. chopped fresh basil
6 c. vegetable stock
1 28-oz. can diced tomatoes
1 15-oz. can cannellini or white beans, drained and rinsed
1 tsp. cumin
1 tsp. sea salt
8 oz. quinoa pasta, seashell or short elbow type
3 T. chopped fresh parsley

1. In a large pan, stir fennel, onion, celery, and olive oil over low heat about 3 minutes.
2. Add garlic, oregano, pepper flakes, and basil, and cook 30 more seconds.
3. Add vegetable stock, tomatoes, beans, cumin, and sea salt.
4. Cook over medium-low heat about 15 minutes, stirring occasionally.
5. Add quinoa pasta and cook over medium heat 10 minutes or until pasta is tender.
6. Garnish with parsley and serve warm.

Carrot Bisque Soup

Cayenne and curry bring out the sweet flavors of the carrots in this flavorful soup.

YIELD: 4–6 SERVINGS

1 medium sweet potato, peeled and cut into small pieces
6 large carrots, peeled and cut into 1/4-inch rounds (approx. 4 c.)
4 c. water
1 medium yellow onion, diced (approx. 1 c.)
2 garlic cloves, minced
2 T. minced fresh ginger
1 T. curry powder
1/8 tsp. cayenne pepper
1 tsp. sea salt
2 T. lime juice
2 c. coconut milk

1. Steam sweet potato and carrots approximately 25 minutes, or until soft and tender.
2. In a large pot cook water, potato, carrots, onion, garlic, ginger, curry powder, cayenne pepper, and sea salt over medium heat 15 minutes.
3. Transfer soup into a food processor or blender and puree until smooth, in batches if necessary.
4. Return pureed soup to pot.
5. Stir in coconut milk and lime juice.
6. Cook over medium-low heat about 5 minutes. Serve hot.

Cauliflower Curry Soup

This curry spice soup gets a welcome tangy sweetness from apple and pure maple syrup.

YIELD: 4–6 SERVINGS

4 c. vegetable stock
1 large head cauliflower, chopped into 1-inch pieces (approx. 6 c.)
1 medium yellow onion, chopped (1 c.)
3 cloves garlic, minced
1 Granny Smith or Pippin apple, peeled, cored, and coarsely chopped (1 c.)
1 T. curry powder
1 T. apple cider vinegar
1 T. maple syrup

1. Simmer vegetable broth, cauliflower, onion, and garlic in a large pot about 20 minutes.
2. Stir in apple and curry powder.
3. Cook over low heat 5 minutes.
4. Let soup mixture cool.
5. Blend mixture in a food processor and blend until smooth.
6. Stir in vinegar and maple syrup.
7. Return soup to pot and cook over medium heat 3 minutes, and serve hot.

Cauliflower Potato Soup

Cooked cauliflower gives this soup a rich and creamy texture.

YIELD: 6–8 SERVINGS

4 heads (bundles) garlic
2 T. extra-virgin olive oil
2 stalks celery, sliced
3 T. thyme leaves, chopped
1 medium yellow onion, diced
1 medium head cauliflower, cut into florets
2 medium russet potatoes, peeled and diced
6 c. vegetable stock
1 tsp. Dijon mustard
1 1/2 tsp. sea salt
1 tsp. black pepper

1. Cut off tops of garlic heads and peel off outer leaves. Steam garlic 5 minutes or until tender.
2. Let garlic cool and squeeze out garlic flesh.
3. In a large pot stir olive oil, celery, thyme leaves, onion, and garlic over low heat about 2 minutes.
4. Add cauliflower, potatoes, vegetable stock, mustard, sea salt, and pepper, and bring to a boil.
5. Reduce heat to a simmer and cook 20 minutes.
6. Let cool.
7. Transfer cooled soup to a food processor or blender and blend until smooth.
8. Return soup to pot.
9. Cook over medium-low heat 5 minutes. Serve hot.

Chilled Cucumber Grape Soup

This is a refreshing twist on a traditional gazpacho.

YIELD: 4 SERVINGS

2 c. vegetable stock
2 large cucumbers, peeled, seeds removed, and sliced
1 jalapeno pepper, seeded and chopped (optional)
6 green onions, sliced
3 stalks celery, sliced
2 Hass avocados
3 T. lime juice
1/4 c. fresh cilantro, chopped
1/4 c. fresh basil, chopped
2 c. seedless green grapes, halved, divided

1. Blend vegetable stock, cucumbers, jalapeno pepper, onions, celery, avocados, lime juice, cilantro, basil, and 1 1/2 c. grapes in a food processor until smooth (or to desired consistency).
2. Stir in remaining 1/2 c. grapes.
3. Refrigerate soup in a 2-quart container about 2 hours or until chilled. Serve cold.

Classic Vegetable Stock

This Classic Vegetable Stock can be used for all the recipes in this book requiring vegetable stock or broth, or you can use vegetable stock purchased at your local supermarket. Low-sodium vegetable stocks can be used in these recipes, also. A great foundation for soups or stews is a flavorful stock that adds welcomed richness to rice dishes, vegetables, and many other savory dishes. Although commercially prepared stocks are readily available, making your own gives you something fresher and is a great way to use leftover vegetables.

When it comes to preparing stock, there is no single recipe. What goes in it will depend on what you have on hand including extra carrot peels and heels, celery tops, and even the skins of onion and garlic. Use our basic recipe for Classic Vegetable Stock as a starting point for experimenting with your own ingredients.

When using root vegetables like carrots, turnips, and parsnips, peeling isn't necessary, just scrub them well. To further elevate the flavor of a basic vegetable stock, try adding dried mushrooms and fresh herbs and spices.

Whenever you prepare fresh vegetables, save the peels and other scraps in a plastic zip-top bag and place them in the freezer, and continue adding to the bag. There's no need to throw out limp carrots or celery stocks that have passed their prime, as they are perfect to add to stock.

Homemade stock is simple to prepare, and it's healthier, more flavorful, and less expensive than most commercial varieties. After making stock, you can portion it into various size containers and store it in the freezer so you can always have vegetable stock on hand.

We use parts of vegetables that may be normally thrown out, such as tops of celery or stalks of broccoli for stock. It's nice to have our own fresh stock to use in soups. However, if you are in a hurry, you can buy organic vegetable stock at most grocery stores. This stock can be refrigerated up to one week.

YIELD: 6 SERVINGS

5 carrots, halved
4 tomatoes, quartered
3 yellow onions, halved
4 celery stalks, with leaves, halved
3 springs of parsley
4 cloves garlic, chopped
2 tsp. sea salt
8 c. water

1. Bring all ingredients to boil in a large stock pot.
2. Reduce heat to low and cover.
3. Simmer one hour.
4. Allow the stock to cool and strain through a fine sieve.

Corn Cashew Chowder

White beans and cashews create a dairy-free, creamy texture for this sweet corn soup.

YIELD: 4 SERVINGS

1 15-oz. can cannellini or white beans, rinsed
1/2 c. raw cashews (soaked 2 hours)
1 large yellow onion, chopped
2 stalks celery, coarsely chopped
1 large russet potato, peeled and cut into 1/2-inch pieces
5 ears corn, kernels removed
4 c. vegetable stock
1 tsp. sea salt

1. Blend cannellini beans and cashews in a blender until creamy.
2. In a large, 4-quart pot, bring bean mixture, onion, celery, potato, corn kernels, vegetable stock, and sea salt to boil.
3. Reduce heat and simmer about 20 minutes. Serve hot.

CHANGE IT UP: Substitute 1/2 c. raw cauliflower for cashews.

Cream of Mushroom Soup

Mushrooms give this soup a hearty, savory, and rich flavor.

YIELD: 4 SERVINGS

3 c. vegetable stock
1/2 c. chopped shitake mushrooms
3/4 c. sliced button mushrooms
1 yellow onion, chopped
2 T. lime juice
1 c. coconut cream
1 tsp. sea salt
1/2 tsp. sage
1/2 tsp. oregano
1/4 tsp. thyme

1. Bring vegetable stock, mushrooms, onion, lime juice, and coconut cream to a boil over medium heat.
2. Reduce heat and add sea salt, sage, oregano, and thyme.
3. Simmer 10 minutes, and serve immediately.

Creamy Tomato Basil Soup

This soup can be served warm or cold.

YIELD: 2 SERVINGS

1 T. extra-virgin olive oil
1 medium yellow onion, chopped
2 cloves garlic, minced
1 tsp. sea salt
1/4 tsp. ground black pepper
1 28-oz. can whole tomatoes
1 c. vegetable stock
1/4 c. chopped fresh basil
1 T. fresh chopped thyme
1 c. almond milk

1. In a 4-quart pot, warm olive oil, onion, and garlic over low heat, and stir about 1 minute.
2. Add sea salt, black pepper, tomatoes (with juice), vegetable broth, basil, and thyme, and bring to a boil.
3. Reduce heat and simmer 10 minutes, stirring occasionally.
4. Stir in almond milk.
5. Blend soup in a food processor or blender until smooth.
6. Return soup to pot, heat, and serve.

Curried Chickpea Soup

Cinnamon and curry add a tantalizing flavor to this chickpea soup.

YIELD: 6–8 SERVINGS

1 T. extra-virgin olive oil
1 c. chopped spinach
1/4 c. chopped cilantro
2 medium tomatoes, chopped
1 yellow onion, chopped
1 T. curry powder
1 tsp. cinnamon
1 tsp. ground turmeric
1/2 tsp. chili powder
1/4 tsp. nutmeg
1 15-oz. can chickpeas
4 c. vegetable stock
1 3/4 c. coconut milk
1/4 c. chopped cilantro, for garnish

1. In a large pot cook olive oil, spinach, cilantro, tomatoes, and onions over medium-low heat 3 minutes, stirring constantly.
2. Stir in curry, cinnamon, turmeric, chili powder, and nutmeg.
3. Continue to cook over low-medium heat 2 minutes.
4. Add chickpeas, vegetable broth, and coconut milk.
5. Cook over low-medium heat 30 minutes. Serve warm, garnished with chopped cilantro.

Fiesta Tortilla Soup

Celebrate the Latin spices in this flavorful soup.

YIELD: 4–6 SERVINGS

2 T. extra-virgin olive oil
1 medium yellow onion, chopped
4 cloves garlic, minced
1 jalapeno pepper, seeded and sliced thinly
1 red bell pepper, seeded and chopped
1 c. corn kernels
6 c. vegetable stock
1 24-oz.can whole tomatoes
1 15-oz. can pinto beans (or 2 c. fresh cooked)
1/2 c. chopped fresh cilantro
1 tsp. sea salt
1/4 tsp. red pepper flakes
1 T. ground cumin
1/2 c. sliced black olives
2 T. lime juice
2 c. baked tortilla chips
1/2 c. diced avocado, for garnish

1. Stir olive oil, onions, garlic, jalapeno, red bell pepper, and corn in a large pot over medium-low heat 1 minute.
2. Add vegetable stock, tomatoes, pinto beans, and cilantro.
3. Stir over medium-low heat 10 minutes.
4. Stir in sea salt, red pepper flakes, cumin, olives, and lime juice.
5. Cook over low-medium heat 5 minutes.
6. Stir in tortilla chips and serve warm, garnished with diced avocado.

Gazpacho

There is nothing like a cold soup on a warm day. This soup is best when the ingredients marinate overnight in the refrigerator.

YIELD: 4–6 SERVINGS

8 fresh plum or heirloom tomatoes, majority of seeds discarded (or 6 canned tomatoes, drained, juices reserved, and roughly chopped)
10 scallions, finely chopped
1 small yellow bell pepper, cored, seeded, and roughly chopped
2 cloves garlic, minced
2 5.5-oz. cans low-sodium tomato juice
1/4 c. tomato paste
1/4 c. extra-virgin olive oil
2 T. red wine vinegar
4 T. freshly squeezed lemon juice
1 1/2 tsp. sea salt
1/4 tsp. cayenne (or more to taste)
1 avocado, sliced in wedges, for garnish
1/4 c. fresh cilantro, for garnish

1. Combine tomatoes, scallions, bell pepper, garlic, tomato juice, tomato paste, oil, vinegar, lemon juice, salt, and cayenne in a bowl.
2. Cover and refrigerate overnight.
3. Transfer half of mixture to a blender and puree to desired consistency.
4. Return soup to bowl and refrigerate until serving time.
5. Garnish with avocado and cilantro leaves, and serve cold.

Minestrone

This minestrone is a hearty meal! Some minestrones add pasta to them. To do so, make 1 cup of your favorite gluten-free pasta, stir in the cooked pasta to the soup, and warm up before serving.

YIELD: 4–6 SERVINGS

2 T. extra-virgin olive oil
1 large onion, chopped
1 leek, sliced
4 cloves garlic, minced
2 zucchini, chopped
2 medium carrots, chopped
1 28-oz. can chopped tomatoes
4 1/2 c. vegetable stock
1 15-oz. can navy or white beans, drained and rinsed
1 large russet potato, cut into about 1/4-inch pieces
3/4 c. shredded green cabbage
1/2 c. green beans, cut into bite-sized pieces
2 T. chopped fresh basil
2 T. chopped fresh parsley
1 c. cooked gluten-free pasta (optional)

1. Cook olive oil, onions, leek, and garlic in a large pot over medium-low heat 2 minutes, stirring constantly.
2. Add zucchini, carrots, and tomatoes.
3. Cook another 2 minutes.
4. Stir in vegetable stock, beans, potato, cabbage, green beans, basil, and parsley.
5. Simmer about 45 minutes.
6. Add pasta, if using, and warm up soup an additional 3 minutes. Serve warm.

Pumpkin Spice Soup

Pumpkin and Yukon potatoes combine to create a creaminess and rich flavor.

YIELD: 4–6 SERVINGS

1 yellow onion, chopped
2 cloves garlic, chopped
2 carrots, sliced
2 celery stalks, diced
4 T. extra-virgin olive oil
8 c. vegetable stock
1 28-oz. can pumpkin puree
6 medium Yukon gold potatoes, peeled and diced
1 tsp. cinnamon
1/2 tsp. nutmeg
1/2 tsp. ground ginger (or 1 T. fresh minced ginger)
1/2 tsp. allspice
3/4 c. pumpkin seeds, for garnish

1. Cook onions, garlic, carrots, celery, and olive oil in a large pot over low-medium heat, stirring, 2 minutes.
2. Add vegetable stock, pumpkin puree, and potatoes, and bring to a boil.
3. Reduce heat and simmer 45 minutes.
4. Stir in cinnamon, nutmeg, ginger, and allspice.
5. Continue to cook over low-medium heat 10 minutes.
6. Let cool.
7. Blend cooled soup in a food processor or blender until smooth.
8. Return soup to the pot and heat over medium heat about 5 minutes.
9. Sprinkle pumpkin seeds on top and serve hot.

Red Pepper and Garlic Soup

Sweet bell pepper infused with garlic makes this a savory favorite soup!

YIELD: 2 SERVINGS

4 heads garlic, peels removed
4 large red bell peppers, seeded and chopped
2 1/2 c. vegetable stock
4 T. sunflower seeds
2 T. chopped fresh basil
1 tsp. sea salt
1/4 tsp. black pepper

1. Steam garlic and red bell pepper about 5 minutes.
2. Blend vegetable stock, garlic, red bell pepper, sunflower seeds, basil, sea salt, and black pepper in a blender until smooth.
3. Warm over medium heat in a medium pot about 5 minutes. Serve warm.

Savoy Cabbage Soup

Savoy cabbage is less pungent than green cabbage and gives this soup a delicate flavor.

YIELD: 4 SERVINGS

3 T. extra-virgin olive oil
1 medium savoy cabbage, shredded
2 stalks celery, sliced
1 yellow onion, chopped
3 cloves garlic, halved
5 c. vegetable stock
1/2 c. brown rice
1 tsp. sea salt
1/2 c. grated vegan mozzarella cheese, for topping (optional)

1. Stir olive oil, cabbage, celery, onion, and garlic and olive oil in a large pot over low-medium heat 3 minutes.
2. Add vegetable stock, rice, and sea salt, and bring to a boil.
3. Reduce heat and simmer about 20 minutes.
4. Garnish with vegan mozzarella cheese shreds, if using, and serve warm.

Spiced Red Lentil Soup

Quinoa is a protein-packed seed found in many gluten-free products because of its grain-like consistency. This seed grows from a plant in the goosefoot family, which also produces edibles such as chard and spinach.

YIELD: 4 SERVINGS

2 T. extra-virgin olive oil
1 large leek, quartered and chopped (1 1/2 c.)
3 cloves garlic, minced
2 c. chopped tomatoes (or 1 15-oz. can chopped tomatoes)
1 red bell pepper, diced
3/4 c. red lentils
1/4 c. quinoa
6 c. vegetable stock
1 tsp. turmeric
1/2 tsp. chili powder
1 tsp. sea salt
1/4 tsp. ground black pepper
2 T. lemon juice

1. Stir olive oil and chopped leeks in a large pot over low heat about 2 minutes.
2. Stir in garlic, tomatoes, red bell pepper, lentils, and quinoa over low heat another 2 minutes.
3. Add vegetable stock and continue to cook, over medium-low heat, 15 minutes.
4. Stir in turmeric, chili powder, sea salt, black pepper, and lemon juice.
5. Cook over medium-low heat 5 minutes, and serve hot.

Spicy Kale Soup

Kale is part of the cruciferous family and contains an antioxidant known as alpha-lipoic acid, which is high in fiber, potassium, vitamin C, and vitamin B6—which are all great for the brain!

YIELD: 4 SERVINGS

2 1/2 c. chopped kale
1/2 c. pumpkin seeds
2 1/2 c. vegetable broth
3 T. lemon juice
1/4 c. apple juice
1 Hass avocado, mashed
1 T. peeled and minced fresh ginger
1 tsp. chili powder
1 1/2 tsp. sea salt
1/4 tsp. black pepper
1/4 tsp. turmeric
1 T. coconut oil
1 T. wheat-free tamari or soy sauce
1 T. fresh cilantro, chopped, for garnish
1/2 c. diced red bell pepper for garnish

1. Blend kale, pumpkin seeds, vegetable stock, lemon juice, apple juice, avocado, ginger, chili powder, sea salt, black pepper, turmeric, coconut oil, and soy sauce in a blender until mixture becomes creamy.
2. Cook mixture in a large pot over medium-low heat 15 minutes, stirring occasionally.
3. Garnish with cilantro and diced red bell pepper, and serve warm.

Spring Green Soup

Add asparagus last in the soup because overcooked asparagus can be a tad stringy. The seasonal flavors of spring come together well in this soup.

YIELD: 4 SERVINGS

1 lb. leeks, diced (4 1/2 c.)
6 green onions, sliced
1 c. diced carrots
2 T. extra-virgin olive oil
5 c. vegetable stock
1 c. sliced green beans
1 c. diced zucchini
1 c. fresh or frozen sweet peas
1 c. sliced asparagus
4 cloves garlic, minced
1 T. chopped parsley
2 T. chopped fresh basil

1. Stir leeks, onions, carrots, and olive oil in a large pot over low heat 3 minutes.
2. Add vegetable stock, and bring to a boil.
3. Reduce heat to a simmer and cook 10 minutes.
4. Add green beans, zucchini, sweet peas, asparagus, garlic, parsley, and basil.
5. Cook over medium heat 15 minutes, and serve warm.

Sun-Dried Tomato and Swiss Chard Soup

Swiss chard, also known as chard, belongs to the same family as beets and spinach. When steamed, this leafy green vegetable adds a pungent flavor to this soup.

YIELD: 6 SERVINGS

2 T. extra-virgin olive oil
1 medium yellow onion, chopped (1 c.)
4 cloves garlic, minced
2 medium carrots, sliced (1 c.)
2 stalks celery, chopped (1/2 c.)
2 c. vegetable broth
2 15-oz. cans diced tomatoes
1 15-oz. can cannellini or white beans, rinsed and drained
1/2 c. chopped fresh basil
1/2 c. sun-dried tomatoes, chopped
1/2 bunch Swiss chard, chopped (approximately 1 c.)

1. Stir olive oil, onion, garlic, carrots, and celery in a large pot over medium-low heat 3 minutes.
2. Add vegetable broth, diced tomatoes, beans, basil, sun-dried tomatoes and Swiss chard, and cook over medium heat 15 minutes.
3. Let cool.
4. Puree cooled soup mixture in a food processor until smooth.
5. Return soup to pot and cook over medium-low heat 5 minutes. Serve warm.

Sweet Beet Soup

Scientists at Wake Forest University and researchers at Translational Science Center found that beets can increase blood flow to area of the brain associated with dementia and improves mental performance. Beets are a good source of potassium and iron, too. When cooking with beets you might want to wear rubber gloves to avoid beet stains.

YIELD: 6 SERVINGS

3 lb. fresh red beets, trimmed, peeled, and cut into pieces
1 large yellow onion, chopped
2 carrots, chopped
1 red bell pepper chopped
2 T. extra-virgin olive oil
2 c. apple juice
2 c. vegetable stock
1 tsp. dried tarragon
1 T. fresh chopped basil (or 1 tsp. dried)
1 tsp. sea salt
1/4 tsp. black pepper

1. Preheat oven to 350 degrees F.
2. In a large bowl toss beets, onion, carrots, and red bell pepper with olive oil.
3. Place vegetable mixture on a baking sheet.
4. Reduce oven temperature to 250 degrees F.
5. Bake 40 minutes.
6. In a large pot, cook apple juice, vegetable stock, and baked vegetables over medium-low heat 10 minutes.
7. Stir in tarragon, basil, sea salt, and black pepper.
8. Let cool.

9. Blend cooled soup in a food processor until smooth.
10. Return to soup to pot and cook over medium heat for 5 minutes. Serve warm.

Sweet Pea Soup

Note that this recipe takes longer because you should soak the peas seven hours before cooking them. Many pea soup recipes use ham; this plant-based version combines the sweet flavors of peas and sweet potatoes and a kick from the chipotle chilies.

YIELD: 6 SERVINGS

1 c. green split peas
2 T. extra-virgin olive oil
2 medium onions, diced (about 3 c.)
4 cloves garlic, minced
1 small green pepper, diced
4 stalks celery, diced (1 c.)
1 large sweet potato, peeled and diced
1 14-oz. can diced tomatoes
1 T. chopped chipotle chili
1 tsp. sea salt
1 tsp. paprika
6 c. water

1. Soak split peas in a large bowl of cold water overnight (about 7 hours).
2. Stir olive oil, onion, garlic, green pepper, and celery in a large pot over low heat about 3 minutes.
3. Add sweet potato, diced tomatoes, chipotle, sea salt, and paprika.
4. Bring 6 c. water and drained peas to a boil in a large pot.
5. Reduce heat to a simmer and cook 1 hour.
6. Add vegetable mixture and cook over low heat 15 minutes. Serve warm.

Tasty Tarragon Pea Soup

Tarragon gives this soup a licorice (anise-y) flavor. This soup can be served warm or cold.

YIELD: 4 SERVINGS

2 T. extra-virgin olive oil
2 medium leeks, white and light green parts thinly sliced (1 1/2 c.)
2 stalks celery, sliced
2 cloves garlic, minced
2 1/2 c. vegetable stock
3 c. fresh or frozen peas
1 T. tarragon leaves, chopped
1/2 tsp. sea salt
1/4 tsp. black pepper

1. Stir olive oil, leeks, celery, and garlic in a large pot over medium-low heat about 2 minutes.
2. Add vegetable stock and peas, and bring to a simmer.
3. Cook for 10 minutes.
4. Remove from heat and let cool.
5. Blend cooled soup and tarragon leaves in a food processor or blender until smooth.
6. Stir in sea salt and pepper.
7. Return soup to pot and heat over medium-low heat 5 minutes. Serve warm.

Via Quinoa Soup

Quinoa is high in protein, fiber, magnesium, and iron. Iron helps increase brain function.

YIELD: 6–8 SERVINGS

3 cloves garlic, minced
1 medium yellow onion, chopped
1 tsp. ground cumin
2 T. extra-virgin olive oil
6 c. vegetable stock
1 large carrot, diced
3/4 c. quinoa, washed and drained
3 c. fresh or frozen corn kernels
1 15-oz. can pinto beans
1/2 c. red bell pepper, diced
1/2 tsp. cayenne pepper
1 tsp. sea salt
1 T. lime juice
1/4 c. chopped cilantro

1. Stir garlic, onions, cumin, and olive oil in a large pot over low heat about 1 minute.
2. Add vegetable stock, carrots, quinoa, corn, beans, red bell pepper, cayenne, and sea salt.
3. Cook over medium-low heat 20 minutes.
4. Stir in lime juice and cilantro, and serve warm.

Watermelon Cucumber Soup

Fresh basil and parsley add wonderful flavors to this sweet and savory chilled soup. Red wine vinegar balances out the sweetness of the melon.

YIELD: 6 SERVINGS

8 c. watermelon (about a 6-lb. watermelon), finely diced
1 medium cucumber, seeded and finely chopped
1/2 c. chopped red bell pepper
1/4 c. fresh basil, chopped
1/4 c. parsley, chopped
3 T. red wine vinegar
2 T. shallots, minced
2 garlic cloves, minced
2 T. extra-virgin olive oil
3/4 tsp. sea salt

1. Mix watermelon, cucumber, bell pepper, basil, parsley, vinegar, shallots, garlic, olive oil, and sea salt in a large bowl.
2. Puree 3 c. of mixture in a blender or food processor until smooth.
3. Transfer into a large bowl.
4. Puree another 3 c. of mixture.
5. Add to smooth soup.
6. Stir in remaining mixture.
7. Refrigerate at least 1 hour to chill before serving.

DELIGHTFUL DESSERTS AND SNACKS

Please note when a recipe calls for unsweetened shredded coconut, you can use reduced-fat unsweetened coconut and still get the same flavor.

When a pie recipe calls for the filling to use cashews, you can either soak the cashews or not. Soaked nuts tend to enhance the nutritional value of the nut.

You can substitute equal amounts maple syrup in any recipe using honey or coconut sugar.

Banana Chia Cookies
Banana Walnut Muffins
Blueberry Bliss Cheesecake
Blueberry Chia Pudding
Blueberry Muffins
Blueberry Watermelon Pops
Carob Fudge Brownies
Cashew Coconut Granola
Chilled Carob Coconut Haystacks
Classic Oatmeal Raisin Cookies
Coconut Macadamia Nut Cookies
Crispy Rice Treats
Double Energy Date Squares
Grain-Free Nutty Granola
Hazelnut Cookies
Lemon Coconut Cheesecake
Lemon Rounds
Lemony Raspberry Bars
Maple Bake-Free Balls
Peanut Butter Cookies
Peanut Butter Dream Pie
Peanut Butter Fudge Pudding
Pear Fig Crisp
Pistachio Cheesecake
Pumpkin Chewy Cookies
Pumpkin Pecan Muffins
Tropical Cobbler
Tropical Fruit Kabobs

Almond Apricot Bites

Dried apricots with almonds make this a sweet and fun treat that can be stored in the refrigerator for up to a week. Soak dried apricots in a little bit of water for 10 minutes to make them softer.

YIELD: 20 BALLS

1 c. almonds
1 c. raisins
1/2 tsp. cinnamon
12 dried apricots (unsulfured), chopped
1/2 c. unsweetened shredded coconut

1. Process almonds, raisins, and cinnamon in a food processor until mixture becomes a smooth, thick almond butter paste.
2. Add chopped apricots and pulse about 30 seconds.
3. Add coconut and pulse another 10 seconds.
4. Scoop out a tablespoon of mixture at a time and roll into balls. Serve room temperature or chilled.

CHANGE IT UP: Substitute cashews for almonds.
Substitute 3/4 c. chopped dates for raisins.

Almond T Cookies

These almond butter cookies are made with teff flour, which gives them a shortbread type of texture. Teff flour is a gluten-free grain that has a mild, nutty flavor. Cookies may look soft when out of oven, but they will firm up as they dry.

YIELD: 35–40 COOKIES

1 1/4 c. teff flour
1/2 tsp. cinnamon
1/2 tsp. aluminum-free baking powder
1/2 c. honey
1/2 c. coconut oil
1 tsp. almond extract
1 c. almond butter
35–40 raw almonds

1. Preheat oven to 350 degrees F.
2. In a large bowl, combine teff flour, cinnamon, and baking powder.

3. In a medium bowl, blend honey, coconut oil, almond extract, and almond butter.
4. Stir wet ingredients into dry mixture, and mix well.
5. Shape dough into walnut-sized balls.
6. Place balls on a baking sheet and gently press an almond on top of each cookie.
7. Reduce oven temperature to 250 degrees F.
8. Bake about 20 minutes.

CHANGE IT UP: Substitute oat flour for teff flour and reduce coconut oil to 1/4 c.
Substitute cashew or sunflower seed butter for almond butter.

Apple Cinnamon Crisp

For this recipe, green apple varieties, such as organic Granny Smith or Pippin, are best to use.

1 c. rolled oats
1 c. oat flour
3/4 c. chopped walnuts
3/4 c. pure maple syrup
1/3 c. sunflower oil
1 T. ground cinnamon
1 tsp. vanilla extract
4 c. unpeeled, diced green apple

1. Preheat oven to 350 degrees F.
2. Lightly oil a 7x11-inch baking dish and set aside.
3. Combine oats, flour, walnuts, maple syrup, oil, cinnamon, and vanilla in a large bowl, and set aside.
4. Place apples in the bottom of the prepared baking pan and cover with oat mixture.
5. Reduce oven temperature to 250 degrees F.
6. Bake for 50 minutes. Serve warm or room temperature.

CHANGE IT UP: Substitute quinoa flakes for rolled oats.
Substitute pecans for walnuts, and add 1/2 c. raisins.

Banana Chia Cookies

This is a moist cookie that tastes best right out of the oven. It makes a terrific breakfast cookie sandwich with sliced bananas and peanut butter. We like to add sunflower seeds to the mixture, as suggested in Change It Up, for a crunchier textured cookie.

YIELD: 20 COOKIES

2 ripe bananas, smashed
1/2 c. unsweetened apple sauce
3/4 c. coconut sugar
1/4 c. chia seeds
1/2 c. oat flour
1 c. rolled oats
1 tsp. cinnamon
1 tsp. vanilla extract
1 tsp. baking powder

1. Preheat oven to 350 degrees F.
2. Place bananas in a large mixing bowl and stir in applesauce, coconut sugar, and chia seeds.
3. Stir in oat flour, oats, cinnamon, vanilla, and baking powder.
4. Place heaping tablespoons of mixture onto a greased cookie sheet.
5. Reduce oven temperature to 250 degrees F.
6. Bake cookies 15–20 minutes. (Cookies will be slightly firm to touch when ready.)

CHANGE IT UP: Add 1/2 c. raw sunflower seeds.

Banana Walnut Muffins

These deliciously moist banana muffins are high in potassium, and walnuts are a rich source of omega-3s.

YIELD: 10–12 MUFFINS

1 1/2 c. oat flour
1/2 c. brown rice flour
2 tsp. baking powder
1 tsp. baking soda
1 tsp. cinnamon
3 ripe bananas, mashed
3/4 c. maple syrup
1/2 c. coconut oil (in liquid state)
1 tsp. vanilla extract
1 c. walnuts, chopped

1. Preheat oven to 350 degrees F.
2. Combine flours, baking powder, baking soda, and cinnamon in a medium bowl.
3. Stir mashed bananas, maple syrup, coconut oil, and vanilla in a large bowl until well blended.

4. Add flour mixture to banana mixture and stir to form a thick batter.
5. Stir in walnuts.
6. Spoon about 2 heaping tablespoons of batter into the cups of a greased or paper-lined standard muffin tin.
7. Reduce oven temperature to 250 degrees.
8. Bake muffins 35 minutes or until a toothpick inserted into the center of a muffin comes out clean.
9. Cool the muffins at least 10 minutes before removing from the tin.

CHANGE IT UP: Sprinkle coconut flakes on top of each muffin.
Substitute 1/3 c. chia seeds or pecans for walnuts.

Blueberry Bliss Cheesecake

Blueberries, cashews, and coconut oil are brain power foods that make this raw, vegan cheesecake full of flavor and so healthy! The cashews can be soaked at least two hours, as soaking raw seeds and nuts bring increases the nutritional value of the nuts. When cutting this, we suggest using a butter knife and gently scooping out the first piece. Then the other pieces will come out easier. We like to place fresh blueberries on top of each slice before serving.

YIELD: 6 SERVINGS

Crust:

2/3 c. almonds
2/3 c. pecans
1/3 c. chopped pitted dates
1 T. water

Filling:

1/2 c. water
1 1/2 c. raw cashews
1/3 c. maple syrup
2 tsp. flaxseed meal
1 tsp. vanilla extract
1/2 c. coconut oil (in liquid state)
1 c. fresh (or frozen) blueberries

1. Grind almonds to a flour consistency in a food processor.
2. Add pecans and dates, and process until dates are completely blended in.
3. Add water, and pulse to combine.
4. Press mixture into the bottom of a 9-inch pan.

5. Refrigerate crust while you make filling.
6. Blend water, cashews, maple syrup, flaxseed meal, and vanilla in a high-speed blender until smooth.
7. Add coconut oil and blueberries, and blend well.
8. Pour filling into chilled crust.
9. Freeze at least 3 hours.
10. Transfer to refrigerator to chill a few hours. Serve cold.

Blueberry Chia Pudding

This pudding requires no cooking and has the delicately sweet flavor of tapioca pudding. Instead of having yogurt, try this pudding with fresh fruit and Cashew Coconut Granola (page 177). We prefer unsweetened almond milk in this recipe.

YIELD: 2 SERVINGS

1 c. dairy-free milk
2 T. coconut sugar
1 tsp. vanilla extract
4 T. chia seeds
1/2 c. blueberries

1. In a small bowl combine milk, coconut sugar, and vanilla.
2. Stir in chia seeds thoroughly.
3. Pour mixture into two glass cups or jars and refrigerate, covered with plastic wrap, overnight, or until pudding reaches the desired thickness, stirring occasionally.
4. Stir in the blueberries or just place a small handful of blueberries on top of the mixture, and serve.

CHANGE IT UP: Substitute raspberries or strawberries for blueberries.
Sprinkle mixed nuts or seeds on top.
Substitute a sliced banana for blueberries.
Substitute maple syrup or honey for coconut sugar.

Blueberry Muffins

Blueberries are our go-to brain fruit! These fluffy muffins have a lightness that practically melts in your mouth.

YIELD: 12 MUFFINS

1 1/4 c. brown rice flour
3/4 c. oat flour
1 tsp. baking soda
1/2 tsp. baking powder
1 tsp. ground cinnamon
3 c. fresh blueberries
1 c. honey (or maple syrup)
1/2 c. almond milk
1/4 c. avocado oil or sunflower seed oil
1 tsp. vanilla extract

1. Preheat oven to 350 degrees F.
2. Combine rice flour, oat flour, baking soda, baking powder, and cinnamon in a medium bowl.
3. Add the blueberries and stir well.
4. Place honey, almond milk, oil, and vanilla in a large bowl and stir until well blended.
5. Add flour mixture to liquid mixture and stir to form a thick batter.
6. Spoon about 2 heaping tablespoons batter into the cups of a greased or paper-lined standard muffin tin.
7. Reduce oven temperature to 250 degrees F.
8. Bake muffins 30 minutes, or until a toothpick inserted into the center of a muffin comes out clean.
9. Cool muffins at least 10 minutes before removing from the tin.

CHANGE IT UP: Add 1/2 c. walnuts, or desired nut or seed.
Add 1/2 c. diced apple.

Blueberry Watermelon Pops

These naturally sweet popsicles are refreshing! Use BPA-free ice popsicle molds (such as Tovolo Groovy Ice Pop Molds; these can be purchased online). To remove the popsicles from molds, briefly run warm water over molds to loosen.

YIELD: 6 POPSICLES

2 c. seedless watermelon, cut into chunks
2 bananas sliced
1/2 c. frozen blueberries

1. Puree watermelon chunks in a blender or food processor.
2. Divide banana and blueberries into six portions.

3. Place portions of fruit into each of six popsicle molds. (Use a popsicle stick to press fruit to bottom.)
4. Fill molds with watermelon puree, place sticks in, and freeze.

CHANGE IT UP: Substitute raspberries for blueberries.

Carob Fudge Brownies

We love carob! Carob is naturally sweet, not bitter like chocolate, and has no caffeine. It's high in fiber and protein, and aids digestion, too.

YIELD: 12 BROWNIES

2 1/2 c. oat flour
3/4 c. carob powder
1 tsp. baking powder
1 3/4 c. honey
3/4 c. water
3/4 c. safflower or sunflower oil
1/2 c. chopped walnuts
1 tsp. vanilla extract

1. Preheat oven to 350 degrees F.
2. Lightly oil a 13x9-inch baking pan and set aside.
3. Combine flour, carob powder, and baking powder in a medium bowl, and set aside.
4. Stir honey, water, oil, pecans, and vanilla in a large mixing bowl until well blended.
5. Add flour mixture to honey mixture, and stir to form a smooth batter.
6. Spoon batter into prepared baking pan and spread in an even layer.
7. Reduce oven temperature to 250 degrees F.
8. Bake 30 minutes or until a toothpick inserted into the middle of brownie comes out clean.
9. Cool at least 10 minutes before cutting into squares and serving.

CHANGE IT UP: Substitute quinoa or rice flour for oat flour.
Substitute hazelnuts, pecans, cashews, or raisins for walnuts.
Substitute macadamia nut oil or coconut oil for sunflower seed oil.
Substitute maple syrup for honey.
Substitute applesauce for oil.

Cashew Coconut Granola

This granola is delicious with non-dairy milk or non-dairy yogurts, with fresh fruit, or as a trail mix for the perfect on-the-go snack. To keep raisins plump, add them to the mixture after it has cooked. Let the granola cool completely before transferring it to an airtight container or plastic zip-top storage bag. Store in pantry up to a week or in the freezer up to 3 months.

YIELD: ABOUT 6 C.

5 c. rolled oats
2 c. unsweetened shredded coconut
1 c. raw cashews
1/4 c. sesame seeds
1 tsp. cinnamon
2/3 c. coconut oil or sunflower seed oil
3/4 c. honey
1 T. vanilla extract
1 c. raisins

1. Preheat oven to 350 degrees F.
2. Stir oats, coconut, cashews, sesame seeds, and cinnamon in a large bowl with a fork.
3. In a medium saucepan cook coconut oil and honey over low heat until well blended.
4. Pour honey mixture over oat mixture and stir well until well coated.
5. Stir in vanilla.
6. Reduce oven temperature to 250 degrees F.
7. Spread mixture on a baking sheet.
8. Bake about 12 minutes, carefully stir mixture with a butter knife or spatula, and bake another 10 minutes.
9. Mix in raisins.

CHANGE IT UP: Add 1/2 c. pumpkin seeds and 10 diced dried figs.

Substitute pistachios, sliced almonds, walnuts, filberts, macadamia nuts, or pecans for cashews.

Substitute honey for maple syrup.

Add 1 T. almond extract and 1/2 c. slivered almonds.

Substitute quinoa flakes or amaranth flakes for rolled oats.

Substitute macadamia nut oil for coconut oil. (There's no need to heat oil to get in a liquid state. Combine this oil with the honey and stir into dry ingredients.)

Chilled Carob Coconut Haystacks

These no-bake, crunchy, sweet balls are a refreshing snack on a hot afternoon. Haystacks are often cocoa, but we like to use carob for a rich, sweet flavor.

YIELD: 14–16 BALLS

3 c. unsweetened coconut, shredded
1/2 c. carob powder
1/2 c. coconut oil
1/2 c. raw honey
1/4 c. almond butter
1 T. vanilla extract

1. In medium mixing bowl combine coconut and carob, stirring well with a fork.
2. In another medium bowl blend coconut oil, honey, and almond butter to make a creamy mixture.
3. Stir coconut mixture into honey mixture.
4. Stir in vanilla extract until mixture becomes moist.
5. Scoop heaping tablespoons and form into 1-inch balls.
6. Place balls on a plate or in a glass container.
7. Refrigerate until chilled, at least 30 minutes.

CHANGE IT UP: Add a ripe mashed banana.

Substitute sunflower seed or peanut butter for almond butter.

Classic Oatmeal Raisin Cookies

A perfect blend of cinnamon and raisins makes this cookie a holiday favorite!

1 1/2 c. oat flour
1 tsp. baking powder
1 T. ground cinnamon
3 c. rolled oats
1 c. raisins
1/2 c. walnuts (optional)
1 c. honey
2/3 c. coconut oil
1 T. vanilla extract

1. Preheat oven to 350 degrees F.
2. Lightly oil a cookie sheet and set aside.
3. Combine flour, baking powder, and cinnamon in a medium bowl.
4. Stir in oats, raisins, and walnuts until well distributed.
5. Blend honey, oil, and vanilla until smooth.
6. Add flour mixture to honey mixture, and stir to form sticky batter-like dough.
7. Drop rounded tablespoons of dough about 2 inches apart on prepared cookie sheet.
8. Reduce oven temperature to 250 degrees F.
9. Bake 15–20 minutes.
10. Cool the cookies a few minutes before removing from cookie sheet. Serve warm.

CHANGE IT UP: Add 1 c. toasted sunflower seeds or unsweetened shredded coconut.

Substitute applesauce for oil.

Coconut Macadamia Nut Cookies

These satisfying cookies are butter free and egg free, and yet they have a rich, delicious "macaroon type" flavor.

YIELD: 30 COOKIES

1 1/4 c. oat flour
1 1/3 c. unsweetened shredded coconut
1/2 c. coconut oil
3/4 c. raw honey
1 tsp. baking powder
1 tsp. vanilla extract
1/2 c. chopped macadamia nuts

1. Preheat oven to 350 degrees F.
2. In a medium bowl stir flour and coconut.
3. In a separate bowl blend coconut oil and honey.
4. Stir flour mixture into honey mixture.
5. Stir in baking powder, vanilla, and macadamia nuts.
6. Place tablespoons of cookie dough onto a cookie sheet, leaving room for the cookies to spread when they cook.
7. Reduce oven temperature to 250 degrees F.
8. Bake 20 minutes.

CHANGE IT UP: Substitute pecans for macadamia nuts.

Crispy Rice Treats

Crispy Rice Treats can be made with any type of nut butter, including sunflower seed butter. We use unsalted peanut butter. Read labels on nut butters to avoid unnecessary ingredients such as sugar, hydrogenated oils, and salt. After cutting these treats into squares, layer in an airtight container for storage. They can be refrigerator up to one week or frozen up to three months. We love to eat these snack frozen, too!

YIELD: 16 2-INCH SQUARES

4 c. crispy brown rice cereal
1/2 c. raisins
3/4 c. raw honey
1 c. peanut butter
1 tsp. vanilla extract

1. Place cereal and raisins in a large bowl.
2. Heat honey and peanut butter in a medium pot over low heat until mixture is well blended and creamy, about 2 minutes.
3. Stir in vanilla and remove from heat.
4. Pour warm mixture into cereal-raisin mixture, and stir well until mixture is well coated.
5. Empty mixture into an 8x11-inch (or 9x9-inch) glass baking dish and spread evenly with a spatula or butter knife. (The mixture is sticky. Use wet hands to place it evenly down.)
6. Refrigerate at least 1 hour or until mixture is firm.
7. With a sharp knife, cut into 2-inch squares.

CHANGE IT UP: Substitute any type of unsulfured dried fruit, such as pineapple, blueberries, mango, apples, and apricots, for raisins.

Add 1/2 c. sunflower seeds, sesame seeds, flaxseeds, chia seeds, or pumpkin.

Add 1/2 c. unsweetened coconut flakes or shreds.

Double Energy Date Squares

Skip the processed granola type bars and grab a Double Energy Date Square. Perfect on-the-go snack or warmed up with vegan sorbet on top. Let these cool before cutting into bars.

YIELD: 12 BARS

1 c. whole pitted dates (about 10 large dates)
1 c. water
4 c. oat flour
4 c. rolled oats
1 T. cinnamon
1/2 c. chopped almonds
3/4 c. sunflower seeds
1 c. coconut oil
1 c. maple syrup
1 tsp. vanilla extract
1/2 tsp. sea salt

1. Preheat oven to 350 degrees F.
2. Soak dates at least 3 hours (or overnight) in water to soften. (Dates will appear to double in size as they fill up with water.)
3. Drain dates.
4. Process drained dates in a food processor until smooth.
5. In a large bowl, mix flour, rolled oats, cinnamon, almonds, and sunflower seeds well.
6. In another bowl, blend coconut oil, maple syrup, vanilla, and sea salt.
7. Add wet ingredients to flour mixture and mix well.
8. Press half of mixture into a greased 13x9-inch baking pan.
9. Spread pureed dates over top.
10. Top with remaining half of flour mixture, and press down lightly.
11. Reduce oven temperature to 250 degrees F.
12. Bake 30–35 minutes.

CHANGE IT UP: Substitute 1 c. dried apricots or black mission figs for dates.

Substitute pecans for sunflower seeds.

Grain-Free Nutty Granola

This nut-infused granola is the perfect snack alone or on top of dairy-free yogurt or milk. We enjoy sprinkling it on Blueberry Chia Pudding (page 174)!

YIELD: 4–6 SERVINGS

1 1/2 c. raw almonds
1 c. raw cashews
1/3 c. raw shelled pumpkin seeds
1/4 c. sunflower seeds
1/2 c. unsweetened coconut flakes
1/3 c. coconut oil
2/3 c. honey
1 tsp. vanilla extract

1. Preheat oven to 350 degrees F.
2. Stir almonds, cashews, pumpkin seeds, sunflower seeds, and coconut flakes in a medium bowl with a fork.
3. Pulse mixed nut mixture a few times in a food processor or blender to break into small chunks.
4. Heat coconut oil, honey, and vanilla in a large saucepan over medium-low heat, allow oil to melt, and stir well.
5. Stir in nut mixture and stir until everything is well coated.
6. Spread mixture onto a baking sheet.
7. Reduce oven temperature to 250 degrees F.
8. Bake 25–30 minutes.
9. Allow granola to cool, and then break into edible pieces.

CHANGE IT UP: Add 1/4 c. flaxseeds to nut mixture.

Add 1/2 c. raisins or favorite dried fruit (chopped) after baking granola.

Add 1 tsp. cinnamon when adding vanilla.

Hazelnut Cookies

These make great dipping cookies and they melt in your mouth! Hazelnuts, also known as filberts, are rich in B vitamins, which are healthful to the nervous system. B vitamins also improve memory and are necessary for the production of neurotransmitters such as serotonin.

YIELD: 20 COOKIES

1/3 c. coconut oil, softened
3/4 c. coconut sugar
1 T. ground flaxseed meal
1 tsp. vanilla extract
2 1/2 c. oat flour
2/3 c. chopped hazelnuts
1 tsp. aluminum-free baking powder
1 tsp. cinnamon
1/4 c. almond milk

1. Preheat oven to 350 degrees F.
2. In a large bowl, blend coconut oil, coconut sugar, flaxseed meal, and vanilla until thoroughly combined.
3. Stir in oat flour, chopped hazelnuts, baking powder, and cinnamon.
4. Add almond milk and mix well.
5. Form heaping tablespoon-sized balls with dough and place on a greased cookie sheet.
6. Reduce oven temperature to 250 degrees F.
7. Bake cookies 15–20 minutes. Cool 5 minutes and serve.

Lemon Coconut Cheesecake

This raw cheesecake is bursting with lemon flavor! The coconut crust complements this tangy pie perfectly.

YIELD: 6–8 SERVINGS

Crust:

2/3 c. almonds
2/3 c. pecans
2 T. unsweetened shredded coconut
1/3 c. organic raisins
1/2 tsp. cinnamon
1 T. water

Filling:

2/3 c. fresh lemon juice
2 c. cashews
1/2 c. maple syrup
2 tsp. flaxseed meal
1 tsp. vanilla extract
1/2 c. coconut oil (in liquid state)

Topping:

1/2 c. shredded coconut

1. Grind almonds to flour consistency in a food processor.
2. Add pecans, coconut, raisins, and cinnamon, and process until raisins are completely broken down.

3. Add water and pulse to combine.
4. Press mixture into the bottom of a 9-inch pan.
5. Refrigerate crust while you make filling.
6. Blend lemon juice, cashews, maple syrup, flaxseed meal, and vanilla in a high-speed blender until smooth.
7. Add coconut oil and blend well.
8. Pour filling into refrigerated crust.
9. Refrigerate pie at least 2 hours.
10. Sprinkle shredded coconut on top and serve chilled.

Lemon Rounds

These lemon balls are full of tangy lemon tartness and are a perfect, quick snack food that can be made ahead of time and kept in the refrigerator. Store in the refrigerator until ready to eat because they will get soft at room temperature if they are out too long. Eat them plain, or roll them in shredded coconut or ground almonds—or both!

YIELD: 24 BALLS

1 1/2 c. almond flour
1/3 c. organic raw coconut flour
1/2 tsp. sea salt
2 T. maple syrup
1/2 c. fresh lemon juice
2 tsp. vanilla extract
1/2 c. coconut oil (in liquid state)
1/4 c. shredded coconut

1. Pulse almond flour, coconut flour, salt, maple syrup, lemon juice, vanilla, and coconut oil in a food processer until well combined.
2. Roll mixture, a spoonful at a time, into a ball shape.
3. Roll balls into shredded coconut.
4. Refrigerate at least 30 minutes, or longer, before eating.

CHANGE IT UP: Substitute 1/2 c. ground almonds or 1/2 c. carob powder for shredded coconut (for rolling).

Substitute 4 pitted dates for maple syrup.

Lemony Raspberry Bars

These bars are free from eggs, butter, white sugar, white flour, and cornstarch, all of which are typical ingredients in a traditional lemon bar. Agar flakes act as a vegan gelatin, giving a wonderful custard consistency to these luscious bars.

YIELD: 12 BARS

Crust:

2 c. rolled oats
1/2 c. coconut oil
2 T. maple syrup
2 T. water
1 T. lemon juice
1 T. vanilla extract

Filling:

1 1/3 c. water
3 T. agar flakes
2/3 c. fresh lemon juice
1 c. raspberries
3 T. arrowroot powder
3/4 c. coconut sugar

1. Preheat oven to 350 degrees F.
2. Lightly grease a 9x13-inch pan.
3. Pulse oats in a food processor about 10 seconds.
4. Add coconut oil and continue to blend an additional 10 seconds.
5. Add maple syrup, water, lemon juice, and vanilla, and pulse until mixture starts to stick together. (Stop periodically and push down the sides with a spatula to help mix ingredients.)
6. Place mixture in prepared pan, patting it down around the pan and pressing it up about 1/4 inch around the pan. (You may need to wet your hands a little to do this.)
7. Reduce oven temperature to 250 degrees F.
8. Bake about 15 minutes.
9. Remove from oven and let crust cool.
10. Let water and agar flakes sit 15 minutes in a medium saucepan.
11. In a small bowl mix arrowroot into lemon juice to dissolve.
12. After the water and agar have sat 15 minutes, bring mixture to a boil.
13. Reduce heat to a simmer and cook 10 minutes or until agar is completely dissolved.
14. Stir in arrowroot-lemon juice mixture, raspberries, and coconut sugar.
15. Simmer 3 more minutes, stirring constantly.
16. Pour filling into prepared crust and let sit about 20 minutes or until it has cooled off.

17. Refrigerate at least 2 hours.
18. Cut into squares and serve.

Maple Bake-Free Balls

These maple bake-free balls have a healthy, nutty crunch. They make a terrific on-the-go snack.

YIELD: 14 BALLS

1 c. Cashew Coconut Granola (page 177)
3/4 c. chopped pecans
2 T. flaxseeds
1 tsp. cinnamon
1/8 tsp. nutmeg
2 T. applesauce
2 T. maple syrup

1. Pulse granola, pecans, flaxseeds, cinnamon, and nutmeg in a food processor until mixture becomes fine.
2. Add applesauce and maple syrup, and pulse until the mixture becomes "doughy" and mixture is moist enough to form balls.
3. Measure out tablespoons of dough and form into balls. (If balls are a bit sticky, then wet fingers and it will make it easier to form balls.)
4. Refrigerate, in a covered container, and serve chilled.

CHANGE IT UP: Substitute 1 c. rolled oats for Cashew Coconut Granola.
Substitute 6 pitted dates for maple syrup.
Add 1/4 c. unsweetened coconut and 1 T. coconut oil.

Peanut Butter Cookies

This melt-in-your-mouth, bursting-with-flavor cookie is one of our favorite snacks.

YIELD: ABOUT 20 COOKIES

2 c. oat flour
1 tsp. baking powder
1 c. pure maple syrup
1 c. unsalted peanut butter
1/3 c. sunflower oil
1 T. vanilla extract

1. Preheat oven to 350 degrees F.
2. Lightly oil a cookie sheet and set aside.

3. Combine flour and baking powder in a medium bowl, and set aside.
4. Stir maple syrup, peanut butter, oil, and vanilla in a large mixing bowl until well blended.
5. Add flour mixture to peanut butter mixture, and stir to form a thick, sticky, batter-like dough.
6. Drop rounded tablespoons of dough about 2 inches apart on the prepared cookie sheet.
7. Reduce oven temperature to 250 degrees F.
8. Bake 15–20 minutes.
9. Cool the cookies on cookie sheet before transferring to a wire rack to finish cooling. Serve warm or at room temperature.

CHANGE IT UP: Substitute sunflower seed butter for peanut butter.

Peanut Butter Dream Pie

This no-bake, raw pie is so easy to make and delicious! It has a fudgy, caramel-y texture. Just before serving, we like to add fresh sliced bananas on top. This pie is easier to cut when you cut it with a butter knife first, and then gently scoop out each pie piece with a spoon or spatula.

YIELD: 6–8 SERVINGS

Crust:

1 c. almonds
7 pitted dates, chopped
2 T. lemon juice
1 T. water
1/2 tsp. ground cinnamon

Filling:

1 1/2 c. raw cashews (soaked at least an hour and drained)
3/4 c. organic, unsweetened, unsalted peanut butter
1/3 c. pure maple syrup
1/3 c. coconut oil
1/4 c. water
1 tsp. vanilla extract

1. Pulse almonds, chopped dates, lemon juice, water, and cinnamon in a food processor a couple of minutes, until mixture is coarse and sticks together.
2. Spoon sections of mixture into a 9-inch pie pan and pat down.
3. Refrigerate crust while you make filling.

4. Pulse cashews, peanut butter, maple syrup, coconut oil, water, and vanilla extract into a food processor until smooth.
5. Scoop mixture into pie crust.
6. Refrigerate at least 1 hour.

Peanut Butter Fudge Pudding

This pudding is easy to prepare. Just don't forget to pop the bananas in the freezer several hours ahead. We use carob powder for a mock chocolaty flavor, but unsweetened cocoa powder can be substituted for the carob. Try the pistachio almond fudge version in Change It Up, as it's a delightful twist on this pudding.

YIELD: 2 SERVINGS

3 frozen bananas
4 dates, chopped
4 T. peanut butter
3 T. unsweetened carob powder
1 tsp. vanilla extract
1/4 c. coconut milk
1/2 c. chopped peanuts
2 strawberries, for garnish

1. Blend banana, dates, peanut butter, carob powder, vanilla, and coconut milk in a high-speed blender or food processor about 30 seconds, until mixture develops a gelato-like consistency.
2. Scoop pudding into two cups, top with roasted peanuts, and place a strawberry on top of each serving.

CHANGE IT UP: Substitute almond butter for peanut butter and pistachios for peanuts, and add 1 tsp. almond extract.

Pear Fig Crisp

Baked pears baked with figs have a delicate, sweet taste that melts in your mouth. This dish can be eaten warm or cold.

YIELD: 12 SERVINGS

Topping:

1 1/2 c. old-fashioned rolled oats
2/3 c. chopped pecans
3/4 c. coconut sugar
1/3 c. oat flour
1 T. ground cinnamon
5 T. coconut oil

Filling:

3 1/2 lb. ripe (or semi-ripe) but firm Anjou pears, peeled and cut into 1/2-inch pieces (approx. 7 pears)
1/2 c. maple syrup
1/2 c. chopped figs
2 T. oat flour
2 T. lemon juice
1 tsp. ginger

1. Preheat oven to 350 degrees F.
2. In large bowl combine oats, pecans, coconut sugar, 1/3 c. flour, and cinnamon.
3. Stir in oil until mixture is evenly moist.
4. In large bowl mix pears, maple syrup, figs, 2 T. flour, lemon juice, and ginger well.
5. Transfer pear mixture into a 9x13-inch baking dish.
6. Sprinkle topping over pears.
7. Reduce oven temperature to 250 degrees F.
8. Bake for about 50 minutes or until pears are tender. Let sit 10 minutes and serve.

CHANGE IT UP: Substitute filberts or sunflower seeds for pecans. Substitute date sugar for coconut sugar.

Pistachio Cheesecake

This raw cheesecake has a smooth, delicate texture and sweet flavor. You can't taste the peas, but they make this pie "pistachio green" while adding nutritional value! This pie is easier to cut with a butter knife, and then gently scoop out each piece with a spoon or spatula.

YIELD: 6–8 SERVINGS

Crust:

2/3 c. almonds
2/3 c. pistachios
1/3 c. organic raisins
1/2 tsp. cinnamon
1 T. water

Filling:

3/4 c. water
1 c. cashews
1/2 c. pistachios
1/2 c. frozen sweet peas
1/3 c. maple syrup
2 tsp. flaxseed meal
1 tsp. vanilla extract
1/2 c. coconut oil (in liquid state)

Topping:

1/2 c. chopped pistachios

1. Grind almonds to flour consistency in a food processor.
2. Add 2/3 c. pistachios, raisins, and cinnamon, and process until raisins are completely broken down.
3. Add water, and pulse to combine.
4. Press mixture into the bottom of a 9-inch pan.
5. Refrigerate crust while you make filling.
6. Blend 3/4 c. water, cashews, 1/2 c. pistachios, frozen peas, maple syrup, flaxseed meal, and vanilla in a high-speed blender until smooth.
7. Add coconut oil, and blend well.
8. Pour filling into chilled crust.
9. Sprinkle pistachios on top of pie.
10. Refrigerate at least 2 hours, and serve chilled.

CHANGE IT UP: Add 1 c. mashed bananas for a banana cheesecake.
Add 1/2 c. carob powder to the filling for a chocolate-y pie.
Add 2 T. shredded coconut to crust.

Pumpkin Chewy Cookies

Maple syrup combined with pumpkin gives this cookie a chewy, sweet flavor. We store these cookies in the freezer (up to four months) just in case we want a quick snack. They taste great frozen!

YIELD: ABOUT 40 COOKIES

2 1/2 c. oat flour
1 tsp. baking powder
1 T. ground cinnamon
1 tsp. ground nutmeg
2/3 c. rolled oats
1 c. raisins
1 c. pumpkin purée
1 c. pure maple syrup
1/2 c. safflower or sunflower oil
1 tsp. vanilla extract

1. Preheat oven to 350 degrees F.
2. Lightly oil a cookie sheet and set aside.
3. Combine flour, baking powder, cinnamon, and nutmeg in a medium bowl.
4. Stir in oats and raisins until well distributed, and set aside.
5. Stir pumpkin puree, maple syrup, oil, and vanilla in a large mixing bowl until well distributed, and set aside.
6. Add flour mixture to pumpkin mixture, and mix well.
7. Place heaping tablespoons of mixture onto prepared cookie sheet at least 2 inches apart, as cookies will spread when heated.
8. Reduce oven temperature to 250 degrees F.
9. Bake 15-20 minutes.
10. Let cookies cool slightly before removing from cookie sheet.

Pumpkin Pecan Muffins

This is one of our favorite muffins! It's moist and delicately sweet, and tastes best right out of the oven!

YIELD: 10 MUFFINS

2/3 c. brown rice flour
1 c. oat flour
2 tsp. cinnamon
1/2 tsp. nutmeg
1 1/2 c. pumpkin puree
1/2 c. safflower oil
3/4 c. honey
1 1/2 T. baking powder
1/2 c. raisins
1/ 2 c. chopped pecans

1. Preheat oven to 350 degrees F.
2. In a medium bowl mix brown rice flour and oat flour with a fork.
3. Stir in cinnamon and nutmeg.
4. Stir in pumpkin puree.
5. While stirring add oil, honey, baking powder, and raisins.
6. Grease muffin tins.
7. Place about 2 heaping tablespoons pumpkin mixture to each tin.
8. Sprinkle pecans on top of each muffin.
9. Reduce oven temperature to 250 degrees F.
10. Bake approximately 30-40 minutes.

CHANGE IT UP: Omit the pecans.

Tropical Cobbler

Pineapples, mangos, and dates create a luscious filling for this tantalizing dessert. Pineapple is high in vitamin B1 and manganese, which promote cognitive functions! This is a real crowd pleaser that is truly unforgettable!

YIELD: 6–8 SERVINGS

Filling:

5 c. fresh pineapple cubes
1/2 c. diced fresh mango
1 c. chopped dates
1 T. vanilla extract
1/2 tsp. cinnamon
1/4 tsp. nutmeg
1/4 tsp. cardamom or allspice

Topping:

1 1/2 c. rolled oats
1/2 c. oat flour
1/2 c. unsweetened pineapple juice
1/4 c. coconut sugar (optional)
2/3 c. chopped macadamia nuts
1 tsp. ground cinnamon
1/4 tsp. cardamom or allspice
1/2 c. macadamia nut oil or coconut oil.

1. Preheat oven to 250 degrees F.
2. Grease an 8-inch-square baking dish.
3. In a medium saucepan stir together pineapple, mango, dates, vanilla, cinnamon, nutmeg, and cardamom.
4. Bring to a boil over medium heat.
5. Cook about 10 minutes, or until dates begin to break apart, stirring frequently.
6. In a large bowl combine oats, flour, juice, coconut sugar, macadamia nuts, cinnamon, and cardamom.
7. Stir in oil.
8. Pour filling into prepared baking dish.
9. Spread oat topping over filling.
10. Bake about 40 minutes. Serve warm or chilled.

CHANGE IT UP: Substitute blueberries for pineapple and raspberries for mango, and substitute unsweetened blueberry juice for pineapple juice.

Add 1/2 c. sunflower seeds to topping.

Substitute 3 c. Grain-Free Nutty Granola (page 182) for entire topping

Tropical Fruit Kabobs

This is a perfect party snack. Kids especially love to grab and eat these colorful kabobs—and they enjoy making them, too!

YIELD: 20 SERVINGS

3 mangos
1 watermelon
1 cantaloupe
1 pineapple
2 papayas
40 green seedless grapes
Toothpicks or skewers

1. Cut mango, watermelon, cantaloupe, and papaya into 1-inch chunks.
2. Place fruit alternately on toothpicks, and serve.

CHANGE IT UP: Add raisins.

APPENDIX A
METRIC CONVERSION TABLES

Common Liquid Conversions

Measurement = Milliliters

1/4 teaspoon = 1.25 milliliters
1/2 teaspoon = 2.50 milliliters
3/4 teaspoon = 3.75 milliliters
1 teaspoon = 5.00 milliliters
1 1/4 teaspoons = 6.25 milliliters
1 1/2 teaspoons = 7.50 milliliters
1 3/4 teaspoons = 8.75 milliliters
2 teaspoons = 10. 0 milliliters
1 tablespoon = 15.0 milliliters
2 tablespoon = 30.0 milliliters

Measurement = Liters

1/4 cup = .06 liters
1/2 cup = .12 liters
3/4 cup = .18 liters
1 cup = .24 liters
1 1/4 cup = .30 liters

1 1/2 cup = .36 liters
2 cups = .48 liters
2 1/2 cups = .60 liters
3 cups = .72 liters
3 1/2 cups = .84 liters
4 cups = .96 liters
4 1/2 cups = 1.08 liters
5 cups = 1.20 liters
5 1/2 cups = 1.32 liters

Converting Fahrenheit to Celsius

Fahrenheit = Celsius

200–205 = 95
220–225 = 105
245–250 = 120
275 = 135
300–305 = 150
325–330 = 165
345–350 = 175
370–375 = 190
400–405 = 205
425–430 = 220
445–450 = 230
470–475 = 245
500 = 260

Conversion Formulas

Liquid

What you know:	Multiply by:	To determine:
Teaspoons	5.0	milliliters
Tablespoons	5. 0	milliliters
Fluid Ounces	30.0	milliliters
Cups	0.24	liters
Pints	0.47	liters
Quarts	0.95	liters

Weight

What you know:	Multiply by:	To determine:
Ounces	28.0	grams
Pounds	0.45	kilograms

APPENDIX B
THE 7-DAY MEMORY DIET MEAL PLAN

Here is a 7-day meal plan that incorporates some of our favorite brain-boosting recipes!

Monday

Breakfast:

Avocado Mango Shake
Tropical Cobbler

Lunch:

Baby Spinach and Pear Salad With Hazelnuts
Cauliflower Potato Soup

Dinner:

Black Bean, Jalapeno, and Cilantro Dip
Polenta Avocado Casserole

Dessert:

Maple Bake-Free Balls

Tuesday

Breakfast:

Blue and Green Tea Smoothie
Blueberry Muffins

Lunch:

Cashew Ginger Rice Salad
Butternut Squash Soup

Dinner:

Fava Bean and Mint Hummus
Springtime Pasta Primavera

Dessert:

Carob Fudge Brownies

Wednesday

Breakfast:

Maui Sunrise Surprise
Coconut Macadamia Nut Cookies

Lunch:

Lemon-Cilantro Chia Slaw
Cream of Mushroom Soup

Dinner:

Great Guacamole
Bueno Bean Tacos

Dessert:

Pistachio Cheesecake

Thursday

Breakfast:

Ginger Pear Smoothie
Double Energy Date Squares

Lunch:

Kale Cashew Salad With Lemon Tahini Dressing
Carrot Bisque Soup

Dinner:

Sage Cannellini Beans With Mushrooms and Hazelnuts
Ginger Mint Spirals With Pine Nuts

Dessert:

Classic Oatmeal Raisin Cookies

Friday

Breakfast:

Green Goddess Smoothie
Lemony Raspberry Bars

Lunch:

Black-Eyed Peas and Tomatoes With Lemon Vinaigrette
Cajun Vegetable Gumbo

Dinner:

Fresh Red Bell Pepper Hummus
Mushroom Lentil Poppers With Cashew-Garlic Sauce

Dessert:

Crispy Rice Treats

Saturday

Breakfast:

Mixed Berry Blast
Grain-Free Nutty Granola

Lunch:

Caesar Salad With Pine Nuts
Creamy Tomato Basil Soup

Dinner:

Eggplant and Olive Dip
Nona's Pizza (including Perfect Pizza Crust and Quick and Easy Tomato Sauce)

Dessert:

Pumpkin Chewy Cookies

Sunday

Breakfast:

Monkey Shake
Peanut Butter Cookies

Lunch:

Cajun Rice and Black Olive Salad
Avocado Gazpacho

Dinner:

Fresh Basil Pesto
Quinoa Walnut Burgers

Dessert:

Banana Chia Cookies

NOTES

Introduction

1. "Dementia." World Health Organization Website, March 2015. Accessed February 17, 2016. *www.who.int/mediacentre/factsheets/fs362/en/#.VqrrtH90EBQ.email.*
2. "A New Case of Dementia Is Diagnosed Every 4 Seconds." 10 Facts on Dementia, World Health Organization Website. Accessed February 17, 2016. *who.int/features/factfiles/dementia/dementia_facts/en/index2.html.*
3. "New MIND Diet May Significantly Protect Against Alzheimer's Disease." Rush University Medical Center Website, March 16, 2015. Accessed February 17, 2016. *www.rush.edu/news/press-releases/new-mind-diet-may-significantly-protect-against-alzheimers-disease.*
4. Paula Cohen. "The MIND Diet: 10 Foods That Fight Alzheimer's (and 5 to Avoid)." CBS News Website, March 30, 2015. Accessed February 17, 2016. *www.cbsnews.com/media/mind-diet-foods-avoid-alzheimers-boost-brain-health/.*
5. Ibid.
6. Weijing Cai, Jaime Uribarri, Li Zhu, Zue Chen, Shobha Swamy, Zhengshan Zhao, Fabrizio Grosjean, Calogera Simonaro, George A. Kuchel, Michal Schnaider-Beeri, Mark Woodward, Gary E. Striker, and Helen Vlassara. "Oral Glycotoxins Are a Modifiable Cause of Dementia and the Metabolic Syndrome in Mice and Humans." *Proceedings of the National Academy of Sciences of the United States of America, volume 111, number 13:* 4940–4945. *www.pnas.org/content/111/13/4940.abstract.*

Chapter 1

1. Interfaith Caregivers Website. Accessed February 17, 2016. *https://interfaithcaregivers.files.wordpress.com.*
2. "Pillar 3: Exercise and Brain Aerobics." Alzheimer's Research & Prevention Foundation Website. Accessed January 12, 2016. *www.alzheimersprevention.org/4-pillars-of-prevention/exercise-and-brain-aerobics.*
3. Gretchen Reynolds. "Can Exercise Reduce Alzheimer's Risk?" Well, *New York Times*, July 2, 2014. Accessed January 12, 2016. *http://well.blogs.nytimes.com/2014/07/02/can-exercise-reduce-alzheimers-risk/?_r=2.*
4. Heidi Godman. "Regular Exercise Changes the Brain to Improve Memory, Thinking Skills—Harvard Health Blog." Harvard Health Blog RSS, 2014. Accessed January 12, 2016. *www.health.harvard.edu/blog/regular-exercise-changes-brain-improve-memory-thinking-skills-201404097110.*
5. "Alzheimer's Disease." Centers for Disease Control and Prevention Website, 2015. Accessed January 12, 2016. *www.cdc.gov/aging/aginginfo/alzheimers.htm.*
6. "Study: Adults Keep Dementia-Related Death at Bay with Exercise." American College of Sports Medicine Website. Accessed January 12, 2016. *www.acsm.org/about-acsm/media-room/news-releases/2012/02/07/study-adults-keep-dementia-related-death-at-bay-with-exercise.*
7. International Table Tennis Federation Website. Accessed February 17, 2016. *www.ittf.com.*
8. "Aerobic Exercise Is as Good for the Older Brain as it Is for the Body." UBC News Website, 2015. Accessed January 12, 2016. *http://news.ubc.ca/2015/07/23/aerobic-exercise-is-as-good-for-the-older-brain-as-it-is-for-the-body/.*
9. "Research Determines How a Single Brain Trauma May Lead to Alzheimer's Disease." Tufts University School of Medicine Website, July 24, 2012. Accessed January 12, 2016. *http://medicine.tufts.edu/TUSM-News/2012/07/Single-Brain-Trauma-May-Lead-to-Alzheimers.*
10. "Music Therapy for Dementia." A Place for Mom Website, April 29, 2015. *www.aplaceformom.com/senior-care-resources/articles/dementia-therapy-and-music.*
11. Ibid.
12. Ibid.

13. Jeff Roberts. "Breakthrough Alzheimer's Treatment Restores Memory." Shift Frequency Website, 2015. Accessed January 12, 2016. *www.shiftfrequency.com/alzheimers-treatment-breakthrough/.*
14. Lisa Mulcahy. "23 Ways to Boost Your Brain." *Parade* Website, 2015. Accessed January 12, 2016. *http://parade.com/426913/lisamulcahy/23-ways-to-boost-your-brain/.*
15. Mayo Clinic Staff. "Dementia." Mayo Clinic Website. Accessed January 12, 2016. *www.mayoclinic.org/diseases-conditions/dementia/basics/prevention/con-20034399.*
16. Dr. Joseph Mercola. "Four Guidelines to Preventing Alzheimer's Disease." Your Medical Detective Website. Accessed January 12, 2016. *www.yourmedicaldetective.com/public/675print.cfm.*
17. Melinda Smith, Lawrence Robinson, and Jeanne Segal. "Alzheimer's and Dementia Prevention: How to Reduce Your Risk and Protect Your Brain as You Age." HelpGuide.org, September 2015. Accessed January 12, 2016. *www.helpguide.org/articles/alzheimers-dementia/alzheimers-and-dementia-prevention.htm.*
18. Kresser, Chris. "Let's Talk About Health." Chris Kresser. February 22, 2013. *http://chriskresser.com*
19. Mulcahy. "23 Ways to Boost Your Brain."
20. "New Study Finds That Closing Your Eyes Boosts Memory Recall." University of Surrey, January 15, 2015. *www.surrey.ac.uk/features/new-study-finds-closing-your-eyes-boosts-memory-recall.*
21. Carol Bradley Bursack. "Vitamins B12, B6 and Folic Acid Shown to Slow Alzheimer's in Study." Health Central Website, May 22, 2013. Accessed January 12, 2016. *www.healthcentral.com/alzheimers/c/62/160989/vitamins-b12-shown-alzheimer/.*
22. Dr. Joseph Mercola. "New Study Confirms Vitamin D Can Improve Brain Disorders including Dementia." Sott.net. Accessed January 12, 2016. *www.sott.net/article/288629-New-study-confirms-Vitamin-D-can-improve-brain-disorders-including-dementia.*
23. Dennis J. Selkoe and Peter J. Lansbury Jr. "Alzheimer's Disease Is the Most Common Neurodegenerative Disorder." National Center for Biotechnology Information Website. Accessed January 12, 2016. *www.ncbi.nlm.nih.gov/books/NBK27944/.*
24. Behnood Abbasi, Masud Kimiagar, Khosro Sadeghniiat, Minoo M. Shirazi, Mehdi Hedayati, and Bahram Rashidkhani. "The Effect of Magnesium Supplementation on Primary Insomnia in Elderly: A Double-Blind Placebo-Controlled Clinical Trial." *Journal of Research*

in Medical Sciences: The Official Journal of Isfahan University of Medical Sciences 17(12) (December 2012): 1161–1169. Accessed January 12, 2016. *www.ncbi.nlm.nih.gov/pmc/articles/PMC3703169/.*

25. Dr. Joseph Mercola. "9 Ways to Improve Your Brain Function." Mercola.com, May 17, 2012. Accessed January 12, 2016. *http://articles.mercola.com/sites/articles/archive/2012/05/17/good-brain-health-tips.aspx.*
26. "Preventing Memory Loss." Harvard Health, June 9, 2009. *www.health.harvard.edu/mind-and-mood/preventing_memory_loss.*
27. Rosick, Dr. Edward R. "Ginkgo Biloba Has Multiple Effects on Alzheimer's Disease." Life Enhancement Website. Accessed January 12, 2016. *www.life-enhancement.com/magazine/article/661-ginkgo-biloba-has-multiple-effects-on-alzheimers-disease.*
28. Dr. Mercola. "The Link Between Alzheimer's, Cinnamon, and Vitamins." Mercola.com, June 13, 2013. *http://articles.mercola.com/sites/articles/archive/2013/06/13/alzheimers-dementia-treatment.aspx.*
29. Lecia Bushak. "How the Probiotics in Yogurt Can Affect Your Mood." Medical Daily, April 11, 2015. *www.medicaldaily.com/mental-health-benefits-probiotics-good-bacteria-may-improve-mood-fight-depression-328882.*
30. "Type 2." American Diabetes Association Website. Accessed January 12, 2016. *www.diabetes.org/diabetes-basics/type-2/.*
31. Erica Kannall. "Why Is Spirulina Good for You?" Healthy Eating, SFGate Website. Accessed January 12, 2016. *http://healthyeating.sfgate.com/spirulina-good-you-6178.html.*
32. Ibid.
33. "20 Common Prescription Drugs That Cause Memory Loss." Eat Local Grown Webiste. Accessed February 17, 2016. *http://eatlocalgrown.com/article/14424-drugs-that-cause-memory-loss.html.*
34. "Americans Being Poisoned Into Psychosis, Violence and Insanity by Prescription Drugs and Heavy Metals." Someone Somewhere blog, November 14, 2015. Accessed January 12, 2016. *https://zedie.wordpress.com/tag/prescription-drugs/.*
35. "Exposure to General Anaesthesia Could Increase the Risk of Dementia in Elderly by 35 Percent." EurekAlert! Accessed January 12, 2016. *www.eurekalert.org/pub_releases/2013-05/eso-etg052913.php.*
36. "20 Common Prescription Drugs That Cause Memory Loss."
37. "Celiac Disease: Fast Facts." Beyondceliac.org. Accessed February 17, 2016. *www.beyondceliac.org/celiac-disease/facts-and-figures.*

38. David Perlmutter, MD. "Grain Brain Describes the Staggering Effects of Carbs on the Brain." Dr. David Perlmutter Website. Accessed January 12, 2016. *www.drperlmutter.com/about/grain-brain-by-david-perlmutter/.*
39. Elaine Schmidt. "This Is Your Brain on Sugar: UCLA Study Shows High-Fructose Diet Sabotages Learning, Memory." UCLA Newsroom, May 15, 2012. *http://newsroom.ucla.edu/releases/this-is-your-brain-on-sugar-ucla-233992.*
40. Ibid.
41. Ibid.
42. Carolyn Gregoire. "This Is What Sugar Does to Your Brain." *The Huffington Post*, April 0, 2015. *www.huffingtonpost.com/2015/04/06/sugar-brain-mental-health_n_6904778.html.*
43. "The Link Between Alzheimer's Disease and Too Much Iron and Copper in the Brain." Examiner.com, August 20, 2013. *www.examiner.com/article/the-link-between-alzheimer-s-disease-and-too-much-iron-and-copper-the-brain.*
44. Melinda Smith, Lawrence Robinson, and Jeanne Segal. "Alzheimer's and Dementia Prevention: How to Reduce Your Risk and Protect Your Brain as You Age."
45. Ibid.

Chapter 2

1. Martha Clare Morris. "Brain Tocopherols Related to Alzheimer's Disease Neuropathology in Humans." Alzheimer's and Dementia. Accessed January 11, 2016. *www.alzheimersanddementia.com/article/S1552-5260(13)02942-7/fulltext.*
2. Catherine Fearte, Cecilia Samieri, Virginie Rondeau, Helene Amieva, Florence Portet, Jean-François Dartigues, Nikolaos Scarmeas, and Pascale Barberger-Gateau. "American Medical Association." *Journal of the American Medical Association VIII, no. 25* (1887): 683.
3. David Perlmutter, MD. "Grain Brain Describes the Staggering Effects of Carbs on the Brain."
4. "New Study Reveals AGEs in Overcooked Food Can Negatively Impact Brain Health | AGE Foundation." AGE Foundation Website. Accessed January 12, 2016. *http://agefoundation.com/new-study-reveals-overcooking-food-can-negatively-impact-brain-health/#.VpSNXkvpVdg.*
5. Cristina Ferrare. "Eating for Your Mind: 10 Healthy Brain Foods." MariaShriver.com, April 1, 2015. Accessed February 17, 2016. *http://*

mariashriver.com/blog/2015/04/eating-for-your-brain-10-healthy-foods-cristina-ferrare/.

6. J. Wang, L. Ho, Z. Zhao, I. Seror, N. Humala, D.L. Dickstein, M. Thiyagarajan, S.S. Percival, S.T. Talcott, and G.M. Pasinetti. "Moderate Consumption of Cabernet Sauvignon Attenuates a Neuropathology in a Mouse Model of Alzheimer's Disease." *The FASEB Journal 20, no. 13* (2006): 2313–320.
7. Suzanne Tyas, PhD. "Alcohol Use and the Risk of Developing Alzheimer's Disease." National Institute on Alcohol Abuse and Alcoholism Website. Accessed February 17, 2016. *http://pubs.niaaa.nih.gov/publications/arh25-4/299-306.htm.*
8. "Explaining How Extra Virgin Olive Oil Protects Against Alzheimer's Disease." ScienceDaily.com, March 20, 2013. Accessed February 17, 2016. *www.sciencedaily.com/releases/2013/03/130320095423.htm.*
9. Andrew Kraft, Xiaoyon Hu, Hyejin Yoon, Qingli Xiao, Yan Wang, So Chon Gil, Jennifer Brown, Ulrika Wilhemsson, Jessica Restivo, John Cirrito, David Holtzman, Jungsu Kim, Milos Pekny, and Jin-Moo Lee. "Attenuating Astrocyte Activation Accelerates Plaque Pathogenesis in APP/PS1 Mice." *Federation of American Societies for Experimental Biology*, October 4, 2012.
10. Anna-Mariya Kirova, Rebecca Bays, and Sarita Lagalwar. "Working Memory and Executive Function Decline Across Normal Aging, Mild Cognitive Impairment, and Alzheimer's Disease." Hundawi Publishing Corporation Website. Accessed January 12, 2016. www.hindawi.com/journals/bmri/2015/748212/.

Chapter 3

1. Thad Godish. "Indoor Environmental Quality." Scribd.com. Accessed January 12, 2016. *www.scribd.com/doc/271305966/Indoor-Environmental-Quality.*
2. "Adoption of Genetically Engineered Crops in the U.S.: Recent Trends in GE Adoption." United States Department of Agriculture Economic Research Service, July 9, 2015. Accessed February 17, 2016. *www.ers.usda.gov/data-products/adoption-of-genetically-engineered-crops-in-the-us/recent-trends-in-ge-adoption.aspx.*
3. Adam Hadhazy. "Think Twice: How the Gut's 'Second Brain' Influences Mood and Well-Being." *Scientific American*, February 12, 2010. *www.scientificamerican.com/article/gut-second-brain/.*

4. Dr. Edward Group. “GMO Foods Cause Gut Damage.” Global Healing Center Website, September 10, 2014. *www.globalhealingcenter.com/natural-health/gmo-foods-cause-gut-damage/.*
5. Ibid.
6. National Center for Biotechnology Information Website. *www.ncbi.nlm.nih.gov/*
7. “Alzheimer’s Disease Education and Referral Center.” National Institute on Aging Website. Accessed February 17, 2016. *www.nia.nih.gov/alzheimers/.*
8. Denise Webb. “Phytochemicals’ Role in Good Health.” September 2013. Accessed January 12, 2016. *Today’s Dietician*, September 2013. *www.todaysdietitian.com/newarchives/090313p70.shtml.*
9. “The American Heart Association’s Diet and Lifestyle Recommendations.” The American Heart Association Website, August 2015. Accessed January 12, 2016. *www.heart.org/HEARTORG/GettingHealthy/NutritionCenter/HealthyEating/The-American-Heart-Associations-Diet-and-Lifestyle-Recommendations_UCM_305855_Article.jsp#.VpV52kvpXR0.*
10. The News Oracle Website. *thenewsoracle.com/.*

RESOURCES

AARP

AARP.org

AARP (originally standing for American Association of Retired Persons) is a membership organization leading positive social change and delivering value to people age 50 and over through information, advocacy, and service.

Alzheimer's Association

www.alz.org

225 North Michigan Ave.
17th Floor
Chicago, IL 60601–7633
(312) 335–8700

Alzheimer's Association of America

www.alzfdn.org

322 Eighth Ave.
7th Floor
New York, New York 10001
(866) AFA–8484

The Alzheimer's Disease Education and Referral Center (ADEAR)

www.alzheimers.nia.nih.gov

P.O. Box 8250
Silver Spring, MD 20907–8250
(301) 495–3311/(800) 438–4380

ADEAR maintains information on Alzheimer's disease research, diagnosis, treatments, clinical trials, and federal government programs and resources. AD Lib, ADEAR's literature database, holds nearly 8,500 materials related to Alzheimer's.

Alzheimer's Disease Centers (ADCs) Directory, National Institutes of Health

Alzheimer's Disease Centers offer diagnosis and medical management; clinical research and drug trials; and information about the disease, services and resources.

Alzheimer's Disease International (ADI)

ADI is an international membership group of Alzheimer's associations. It also provides information in several languages, statistics on the number of people with dementia worldwide, and the implications for the distribution of research funding, especially in developing countries.

Alzheimer's Research Forum

This site reports on the latest scientific findings, from basic research to clinical trials; creates and maintains public databases of essential research data and reagents; and produces discussion forums that can contribute to the global effort to cure Alzheimer's disease.

Alzheimer's Foundation of America

www.alzfdn.org
(866) AFA–8484
care ADvantage magazine
www.afacareadvantage.org
(888) AFA–8484

Centers for Disease Control and Prevention

www.cdc.gov
(800) 311–3435

Centers for Medicare & Medicaid Services

www.cms.hhs.gov
(800) MEDICARE

Children of Aging Parents

www.caps4caregivers.org
P.O. Box 167
Richboro, PA 18954
(800) 227–7294

Clinicaltrials.gov

ClinicalTrials.gov
This registry lists federally and privately supported clinical trials conducted in the United States and around the world.

Dementia Education & Training Program (For Physicians)

www.alzbrain.org/prevention.cgi?pg=physician
(800) 457–5679

Falls Free Coalition

www.healthyagingprograms.com
(202) 479–1200

Family Caregiver Alliance

www.caregiver.org
180 Montgomery St.
Suite 1100
San Francisco, CA 94104
(800) 445–8106

MedlinePlus Health Information

www.nlm.nih.gov/medlineplus/
This Website lists generic and brand names, precautions, and side effects for more than 9,000 prescription and over-the-counter drugs.

National Family Caregivers Association

www.thefamilycaregiver.org
10400 Connecticut Ave.
Suite 500
Kensington, MD 20895–3944
(301) 942–6430/(800) 896–3650

National Institute on Aging

www.nia.nih.gov
(800) 222–2225

National Institutes of Health

www.clinicaltrials.gov
(301) 496–4000

Partnership to Fight Chronic Disease

www.fightchronicdisease.org

A Place for Mom

www.aplaceformom.com
A Place for Mom connects moms, dads, seniors, and families looking for eldercare, from finding the right nursing home, dementia care, or assisted living to researching VA benefits and how to pay for senior care.

The President's Council on Physical Fitness and Sports

www.fitness.gov
(202) 690–9000

PubMed

www.ncbi.nlm.nih.gov/pubmed
A database of more than 19 million citations for biomedical literature, life-science journals, and online books.

ResearchMatch

www.researchmatch.org
A free and secure web-based clinical research registry that connects people who want to participate in clinical studies with researchers who are seeking volunteers.

INDEX

ABOUT THE AUTHORS

Judi and Shari Zucker: The Double Energy Twins

Judi and Shari Zucker began their joint writing career when they were still in high school. Eating nutritious, plant-based, whole foods gave them the energy they needed to break the women's one- and two-mile track records at Beverly Hills High School—records that still stand today. Having all that energy inspired them to share the secrets to their success, which led to the publication of their first book, *How to Survive Snack Attacks—Naturally*, in 1979 when they were just 17 years old. This was soon followed by *How to Eat Without Meat—Naturally* in 1981, *Double Your Energy With Half the Effort* in 1991, *The Double Energy Diet*] in 2008, *The Ultimate Allergy-Free Snack Cookbook* in 2011 (Square One Publishers), and *The Ultimate Allergy-Free Cookbook* in 2015 (Square One Publishers).

Both Judi and Shari graduated from the University of California at Santa Barbara with degrees in ergonomics (the study of human physiology, physical education, and nutrition) and went on to serve as media specialists for General Mills, promoting and demonstrating Nature Valley Granola products on a six-week media tour titled "Snack Sense." In spring 2009 they signed an endorsement deal with derma e natural skincare products, as they truly believe in taking care of one's body inside and out. Judi and Shari currently do cooking demonstrations for eHow and lecture at the University of California, Santa Barbara (UCSB) for their health and wellness program.

Following the publication of their earlier books they appeared on both local and national television talk shows, including *Hour Magazine*, *Regis Philbin*, and *AM Los Angeles* as well as national shows such as *TODAY*, *Home & Family*, and *The Better Show*. Judi and Shari are in the process of packaging and marketing their own "Zookie Cookie," a delectably wholesome morsel that developed from a closely guarded recipe.

Shari is married to Daniel Kilstofte, owner of a high-tech company, and they have twin sons, Max and Miles (the fifth straight generation of twins in the Zucker family!), and a daughter, Mattea. Judi is married to Chris Mjelde, a dentist, and they have a daughter, Taryn, and a son, Tanner. Both Judi and Shari live in Santa Barbara, California.